Beyond the Bump

A clinical psychologist's guide to
navigating the mental, emotional and
physical turmoil of becoming a mother

Beyond the Bump

SALLY SHEPHERD

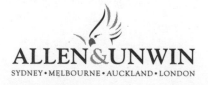

ALLEN&UNWIN

SYDNEY · MELBOURNE · AUCKLAND · LONDON

Allen & Unwin
83 Alexander Street
Crows Nest NSW 2065
Australia
Phone: (61 2) 8425 0100
Email: info@allenandunwin.com
Web: www.allenandunwin.com

 A catalogue record for this book is available from the National Library of Australia

ISBN 978 1 76052 999 4

Pages 43, 230–1: extracts from the book *The Power of Now*. Copyright © 2004 by Eckhart Tolle. Reprinted with permission by New World Library, Novato, CA. www.newworldlibrary.com.

Page 208: material from G.D. Chapman, *The 5 Love Languages: The secret to love that lasts*, Chicago: Northfield Pub, 2010, reproduced with permission.

Index by Puddingburn
Set in 13.1/18.5 pt Garamond Premier Pro by Midland Typesetters, Australia
Printed and bound in Australia by Griffin Press, part of Ovato

10 9 8 7 6 5 4 3 2 1

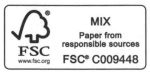

For my darling son, Eliah, my husband and best friend, Gavin, and my wonderful parents, John and Linda. Your guidance, love and support carried me through.

And for all mums everywhere—may we lift each other up, always.

Contents

Introduction

While I was pregnant I attended prenatal appointments with my local midwives. They were lovely, angels incarnate. They made me less terrified of the whole 'bringing forth a human life into the world' thing (still a bit terrified, naturally). But they kept asking me to make a 'birth plan'. It is what it sounds like: my plan for the birth of my son.

'Hey,' I said, 'isn't that *your* job? I'm nowhere near as experienced'—a diplomatic way of saying I have no idea what I'm doing. My sarcasm and awesome joke were not appreciated, and they sent me home to think about what I wanted out of the birth, aside from a brand new, real live human being to take home!

I didn't make a birth plan. I started to but ended up staring blankly at a piece of paper for about half an hour, eventually writing down (and then crossing out because I felt like an idiot with poor priorities), 'bring snacks'. I ultimately planned to have a baby and leave the how up to the professionals. As it turned out, my son was born five weeks early (as impatient then as he is now, over three years later) so I thought I'd gotten away with it, until I had my first contraction, felt an unholy amount of pain, and realised that there was no chocolate in sight. Not so smart now are you, Miss 'I don't need a plan!'

In hindsight, had I made an elaborate (read: any) plan there was no guarantee that it would have worked out. During the first few months of my son's life, nothing at all went to plan! Even the plans that I did make went to hell in a figurative handbasket, because the truth was, I was so completely unprepared for what having a newborn would be like. I had read one book on birthing a baby and exactly nothing on *parenting* said baby from now on. This is hard for me to admit—even embarrassing as I am a clinical psychologist—because I usually pride myself on research, thoughtfully considered plans, and getting things 'right'.

Seven months straight of nausea, vomiting, insomnia, pain, and foggy-minded fatigue probably didn't help with the whole 'getting prepared' thing. It's cruelly ironic that we're expected to get ready for one of the biggest transitions of our lives during the same time period where one day, as I did, you might just get in the car to go and buy milk and forget to put on pants. But also, I just assumed we (my husband and I) would be all right. Everyone else, it seemed, had done it before us and been fine. How hard could it be? Spoiler alert: very.

You may be getting the picture that I struggled with the newborn stage. I don't mean to make it sound like having a newborn at home is awful. Scratch that—yes, I do, because it is sometimes. It is wonderful and terrible simultaneously.

It was a time when I was never alone, but always lonely. I was desperately, scarily tired, but unable to rest. Always busy, but never accomplishing anything. I was completely bored, but unable to concentrate. It was a time when I was overburdened with new responsibilities yet had no control over anything.

It's also a joyful, mesmerising, mind-blowing, surreal, funny, fun and special time. Above all, it is a *major* life change that requires significant adjustment. I didn't realise how much it would change everything about my life. My husband and I had been together for thirteen years before our son was born, so we were used to our life. We knew what we liked and we liked what we knew. That cosy, familiar routine changed dramatically after our son was born.

Knowing what to expect is so, so, so—I could write 'so' a hundred more times and it would still not be enough—vitally important. Do as I say, not as I do, right? It's like tripping over a shoelace. If we pretend it's not happening we might land flat on our faces. If we accept what is coming, we'll hopefully put out our hands and steady ourselves.

Research consistently shows that having realistic expectations prior to a drastic life change helps people to adapt and adjust to the 'new normal'. If our expectations are unrealistic, idealised, or even non-existent, it can really hinder our adjustment process, making it an uphill battle to adapt—in this case, to our new role as 'mum'. In some cases, it can even contribute to significant postpartum mental health difficulties like postpartum depression and anxiety.[1]

My own expectations were not realistic. Some were idealised, dreamy impressions that I probably picked up from movies and books. Some things I hadn't thought about much at all. Some of my expectations were downright weird.

In the process of writing this book, I have spoken to many, many mums (and some dads too). What a relief, but also a surprise, to discover that many of them had felt the same way as me! Maybe, just maybe, I was normal after all. Who would have thought?

Here are some of the unrealistic and idealised expectations I, and others, have fessed up to having:

- Life as I know it will stay the same. I don't want to be one of those people who make life all about their kids. Baby can just fit in to my life as it is now. *Um, no. Not really.*
- Parenthood is natural. I'll just know what to do when the time comes. *To a certain extent it is intuitive, and I surprised myself with some of the things I did just 'know' but it is also a demanding job and necessitates a lot of learning and new skills.*
- Babies are super cute. *Ha. Not all the time, my friend. Not all the time* *thinks back darkly to one particularly memorable 2 a.m. simultaneous poo/vomit explosion*.
- Breastfeeding will come naturally because it is a natural process. *Not always.*
- I will fall in love and bond with my baby from the beginning. *Again, not always.*

Of course, there are lots more where those came from but if I tried to list them all I'd be here all day—and I've got a book to get on with writing!

My (somewhat lofty) goal here is for women to be able to access in one place a bunch of information, backed by science and reflected in real experiences, about what it can be like to suddenly become 'mum'. I want to discuss the common challenges that mums experience during their first year postpartum. Because we know that realistic expectations and being prepared help us to adapt and adjust to life changes, I hope this will help to set you up on a smoother transition to motherhood.

I want to make it really clear that, while I have focused on the common challenges faced during the adjustment to parenthood, having a baby is not all chaotic days, sleepless nights, cracked nipples and poo explosions. This book is concerned with the challenges, because the challenges seem to be what lack discussion in society. I talk about realistic expectations, but I don't equate 'realistic' with 'negative'. I don't mean to say that you should *only* expect the first year to be challenging. It is realistic to expect the amazing alongside the . . . well . . . not so amazing.

I've done a lot of research into the adjustment to parenthood. (Gosh, wouldn't that have been handy *before* I became a mum—twenty–twenty hindsight and all that?) I discovered that, indeed, the research does indicate the newborn period and the transition from child-free to parenthood has a major effect on people's psychological health and well-being. There is a significant body of research from the last 50 years on this, some early researchers even referring to new parenthood as a 'crisis'. This effect has been found to be greatest for women, and this (as well as the fact that

I am one) is why I am primarily writing for new mums, although I am sure dads face several of the same issues.

As well as the research, I reflect on my own experiences, and most importantly, I've spoken to dozens of other women about their experiences of early motherhood—their names have all been changed in this book to protect their privacy and confidentiality. Of course, every mum and every baby are individuals, so you may have struggled in an area that I've not considered. You may identify with some or all of the areas I've included.

On that note, I know you are super busy looking after your contribution to the species, so I've written each chapter so that it stands alone and discusses one specific challenge. You can read it gradually, taking as much time as you need to pay most attention to what's relevant to you. And feel free to read the chapters in any order you want to, or skip those that you think aren't relevant to you.

The chapters all flow the same way. I've started each with a discussion of the area of focus, what the research says about it, and what my own experiences have been. I go on to a section called 'Her story', which consists of a story, or stories, of women who have experienced that topic. I then go on to discuss ideas and possible strategies in a section called 'Let's Get Practical'. Here I ask you to do some work! There are reflection questions and/or activities, and you may like to have a journal dedicated to doing these. Writing can be a cathartic, freeing experience. Sometimes I don't even realise I am thinking something until I get it down onto paper!

I want to make it clear, though, that this book isn't meant to replace the advice of your personal healthcare team. It is an overview of common challenges faced in the postpartum period, and it is intended to normalise, raise awareness and lead you towards healing and seeking help if it is required. If you are struggling, speak to a GP or a therapist. Postpartum adjustment and mental health issues can be so deep and complex, and it is not within the scope of this book to be able to dig as deep into your personal situation as you may need to.

Whether you are trying to conceive, are pregnant, a new mum, or a mum expecting another child, my biggest hope is that my words can help to let you know that *you've got this, mama.* You are getting prepared. (Just the fact that you have chosen to pick up this book is evidence of that!) You are not alone.

We are, in many ways, all in the same boat—sometimes hanging off the side, barely gripping on with one badly manicured fingernail and treading water with the other hand, but together nonetheless. If you are one of those people treading water right now, please reach out to someone you trust. You deserve it, and so does your baby. A healthy and happy mum is their most important asset!

Let's get started!

1

On Pregnancy: The good, the bad and the ugly

Trying to conceive

My husband and I were together for thirteen years before I fell pregnant with our son. But what most people didn't know was that this wasn't through a lack of trying. Having a baby first entered our minds around four years prior to his birth. I remember that day like it was yesterday. We went for a long walk on the beach at sunset—*yes, really!*—and decided we were ready to start trying. This was a big deal to us, a couple who wasn't convinced they would ever have kids. We still felt like we *were* kids. (We absolutely weren't, but denial is a beautiful thing!) That night felt like a momentous occasion as I tossed my pill packet in the bin and prepared to begin the epic journey of parenthood.

And then . . . nothing.

Nothing, nothing and then more nothing. How anticlimactic!

Every month, *for years*, the days between ovulation and my period—the dreaded two-week wait—were a source of stress. Lots of months I was *sure* I was pregnant, and even felt the 'signs'—sore breasts, nausea, tiredness—only to discover that it was 'all in my head' when my period arrived, on time as always, predictable as a bee in a hive.

We didn't tell people we were trying to have a baby. We'd already been married for a long time so we were asked *a lot* about our reproductive plans. Some comments stung more than others. 'You don't know real love until you've had a baby' was among the worst.

I don't really know why we didn't want to tell anyone. Perhaps it was the fear that we would never be able to conceive and that we'd have a lifetime of people fruitlessly assessing me for pregnancy symptoms and giving me the side-eye when I drank water at a wedding. Maybe it was just embarrassing. ('Hey there, I'm going to be having regular, unprotected sex and peeing on plastic objects for a while now—what's going on with you?') There were also a lot of women in my circle of friends and family getting pregnant, and I didn't want them to dread sharing their joy with us. Whatever the reasons, no one knew we were trying. It was a long, uncertain and lonely period, that at the same time felt sort of golden, like my husband and I had a secret hope blazing within us individually and as a couple. I wasn't in a rush to get pregnant so much as I was in a rush just to *know that I could*.

Up to one in six Australian couples experience infertility—the inability to fall pregnant after a year or more of trying to—but I felt like we were the only ones. We weren't telling anyone, so I could only assume other people I knew were going through it alone too. I've since found out that that was indeed the case. The loneliness of watching other people's dreams come true, sharing their dreams but not sharing our dreams *with* them, was crippling some days. But still, you keep smiling. Keep trying. Keep hoping.

Pregnancy

I was *stunned* when I finally saw that long-yearned-for second line on the pregnancy test. It was a sight I'd coveted every month for long enough that I truly thought it would never happen. Finally, it was our time! I harboured images of myself glowing, peacefully looking out of my kitchen window as the mild breeze softly rippled through the lace curtains, as I dreamily rubbed my perfectly rounded belly. (The rest of me still super svelte, of course.) That didn't happen. For one thing, I don't own any lace curtains, and also, I think I was getting a mental image from my memory of an old nursing mothers' booklet my mum had lying around the house when I was little—I think the lady (on the booklet, *not* my mum) was a cartoon. Plus, I was never super-svelte to begin with.

Almost immediately, the nausea and vomiting started. Up to 90 per cent of pregnant women get some form of morning sickness, so I didn't feel particularly special, just sick. But it didn't end until some time after I had given birth—I was vomiting in the shower while my husband held our new baby! I always thought morning sickness stopped after around week 12 of pregnancy; or at the very least, *surely after you'd given birth!* Apparently, this is not always the case, although for many women it does get a lot better after the first trimester has passed—I just wasn't one of them.

Vomit wasn't the only form of bodily fluid being expelled in copious quantities by my rapidly expanding pregnant body, either. I learned early on—the hard way—that I could not simply vomit into the toilet, nor could I simply go to the toilet for an *ahem* bowel movement. One evacuation did not occur without the other, and so my bathroom visits were executed with a thoughtfully planned proficiency—specifically, I used a bucket *and* the toilet simultaneously. Every time. Yes, I was glowing, even if glowing meant tear-stained, red-faced and sweating profusely.

My 'morning sickness' lasted all day, every day. It also lasted for my entire pregnancy and then some. At the same time as I hated it, I also saw it as a comfort, a friend, an assurance that I was in fact still pregnant.

I was terrified for my entire pregnancy that we would lose the baby. We had tried for so long, and it could have been over so quickly. I knew the statistics—up to one in four confirmed pregnancies end in miscarriage; and, as more women miscarry before they even know they are pregnant, the stats are probably even higher. People don't talk about it much, but it happens all the time. I didn't see my fear as irrational, because I knew it happened to lots of people: even people we know, whether we knew about it happening or not.

My fears were made a million times worse when I began to bleed regularly throughout pregnancy. My first big bleed was during early pregnancy. It was just like a normal period and

I was positive that my baby had died. I had an ultrasound scan, expecting the worst, only to be surprised with the best news possible: my baby was fine. But it kept happening. Every month like clockwork, just like my ever-reliable period, I would bleed. Every time I went to the toilet I would practically pull out a magnifying glass to analyse the contents of the toilet paper, searching for tinges of pink. I would pretend I needed to go to the toilet, just so I could check again. (I went through so much toilet paper during this time I should have bought stocks in Sorbent!) Even though every month it was fine, I continued to fret and to expect the worst.

I never found out why I was bleeding. The doctors said that sometimes it just happens. I researched it *a lot* during pregnancy, as you can imagine. I found out that up to one in four women experience bleeding during pregnancy, and many of them go on to give birth to a healthy baby. However, it is always a good idea to be checked out by a doctor if you experience any type of bleeding during pregnancy. It can be a sign of miscarriage, but it can also be due to implantation of the embryo into the uterus, cervical changes, intercourse or infection.

It was the opacity of pregnancy that I disliked the most. I wished that pregnant bellies came with a glass panel. (Bit of a design flaw there.) In between ultrasound scans there is no way of knowing if your baby is okay. I bought a foetal doppler online for $30, but I didn't really know how it worked. I would swish it around my belly for a while until I heard something that sounded like horses galloping, as advised. But I had no real idea about what that sound was—it could have been my lunch digesting—so it was of little comfort.

I became so ridiculously anxious during pregnancy that, as much as I'm ashamed to admit it, I felt relieved when my son was born early. Even though I knew it was a risk for him to be premature, I just wanted him out where I could see him, where I could count his fingers and toes.

Her story: Jasmine

Jasmine was 29 years old when she found out she was pregnant. She had been trying to conceive for seven months, and she and her partner were over the moon when they discovered that they were 'Pregnant: 2–3 weeks', as their digital pregnancy test told them. Jasmine had noticed a small amount of bleeding, more 'spotting', a few days before her period would normally arrive. She furiously googled this and found out that it could have been something called 'Implantation Bleeding', which she learned is basically the embryo implanting itself into the uterus lining. She was still worried though, and contacted her GP, who referred her for a 'dating scan'—an early ultrasound to see how her pregnancy was going.

Jasmine also had a series of blood tests to assess her hormone levels. They were rising, but not as much as they should have been.

By the time she got to her ultrasound scan, Jasmine said she was resigned to the fact that she may not be getting good news. She didn't. When she should have been around nine weeks pregnant, according to the dates of her last period, her baby was around the size of a six-week-old embryo, and it didn't have a heartbeat. There was still some hope, the doctor advised her, because maybe her dates were wrong, and if they were wrong then it may still have been too early to detect a heartbeat.

She went back the following week—the longest seven days ever—for a follow-up scan. Again, the news wasn't good: there was still no heartbeat. A few weeks later, Jasmine's body still thought it was pregnant, although the embryo had died weeks ago—this is called a 'missed' or 'silent' miscarriage—so Jasmine needed to go to hospital to undergo a procedure called a dilation and curettage to remove the pregnancy tissue to prevent infection and maybe even future infertility.

Two months after the procedure, Jasmine fell pregnant again quickly. She went on to give birth to a healthy baby boy. She still feels a pang when the date that could have been her first baby's birthday passes, two months before her son's, and she feels some inner conflict that if her first baby hadn't died, then she wouldn't have had her second. She doesn't know what to do with this thought when it appears.

Her story: Rebekah

Rebekah fell pregnant on her third month of trying. She felt incredibly blessed and thrilled when she found out the good news. She did *five* pregnancy tests, because she couldn't believe it had happened so fast! A couple of weeks later she began to feel sick, and not just a little bit. She remembers her first 'big vomit'—it went all over her feet in the shower. She said she didn't have the will to keep standing up after that, so she got out of the shower without even properly washing her feet. Lying in her bed, the smell triggered another bout of vomiting, which she laid in for an extra half an hour before she felt able to get up.

Rebekah remembers vomiting into an empty coffee cup in her car, into a pot plant in her office, and in the gutter on the side of the road. Some days she vomited up to ten times! She was losing weight, dehydrated, and then her vomit started coming up with streaks of blood. She tried everything—anti-nausea medications, injections, bed rest, drips. Nothing worked. She was then diagnosed with hyperemesis gravidarum (HG), a form of extremely severe and persistent 'morning' sickness.

Rebekah says that her HG lasted all the way through her pregnancy and didn't cease until around three days after she had given birth. Her HG made it hard for her to enjoy any part of being pregnant, but Rebekah says that her daughter is totally worth every vomit-filled day—most of the time.

Let's get practical

In these sections, I'll provide you with possible tips and ideas for coping with the common challenges we discuss in each chapter. Some may be more relevant to you than others, so feel free to take on board only the advice that suits you, and to seek medical advice regarding any ideas that you choose to use. I hope that the following strategies will help you navigate conception and pregnancy. Peoples' experiences throughout this stage are so varied. It can be heartbreaking, confusing, overwhelming, physically draining, exciting, peaceful or scary. Or any combination of the above!

Find your online tribe

If, like me, you are hesitant to tell people that you are trying to conceive, or if you are looking for people at the same stage of pregnancy as you, there are excellent places online to chat to other women in your position. There is a beautiful, thriving community of mums and mums-to-be at www.babycenter.com.au and other sites, and newcomers are always welcome. There are groups for infertility, for conception, for loss, for pregnancies with babies due every month of the year. Lots of women I spoke to found long-term friends out of these types of online groups.

To help you out when online, here is a list of the acronyms commonly used in mum forums. I had no idea what anyone was talking about during my first few months on these forums, so this might save you the mental gymnastics I went through. You're welcome!

NAVIGATING ONLINE ACRONYMS OF CONCEPTION AND PREGNANCY

AC	Assisted conception
AI	Artificial insemination
BBT	Basal body temperature
BC	Birth control
BFP/BFN	Big fat positive or big fat negative (as in, on a pregnancy test)

CM	Cervical mucus
DD/DS	Dear daughter/dear son
DPO	Days past ovulation
DTD	Do the deed (yes, as in sex)
FTM	First-time mum
HPT	Home pregnancy test
IVF	In vitro fertilisation
LO	Little one
LP	Luteal phase
MC	Miscarriage
MMC	Missed miscarriage
MS	Morning sickness
NTNP	Not trying, not preventing (as in, pregnancy)
OH	Other half
OPK	Ovulation predictor test kit
OWT	Old wives' tale
POAS	Pee on a stick (as in, pregnancy test)
TTC	Trying to conceive
US	Ultrasound
VBAC	Vaginal birth after caesarean

Deciding when to tell

You find out you are pregnant: now for the big reveal!

Most people wait until they are 12 weeks pregnant to tell society at large—and write the obligatory social media post, of course. This is usually because around that time the risk of miscarriage drops significantly. It doesn't drop to zero per cent but it does become much less likely, especially if you have already had an ultrasound and seen your baby's heartbeat.

It is unquestionably less complicated to deal with the world after a miscarriage if no one knows you have been through one. However, the risk, if no one knows you were pregnant, is that you may find yourself without much-needed support in the event of a miscarriage. You may also lack support while going through morning sickness, anxiety and fatigue during your first few weeks or trimester. So you may consider telling a few select people earlier than the 12-week mark—people who you would like to be part of your support system if you did in fact miscarry. This might include a parent, your best friend, even your boss (if you feel comfortable).

Everyone will feel differently about this, though, so do what feels right for you.

Simplify your life

If ever there was a time to not have to 'do it all' it is now. You are already charged with the task of building an entire human. If you don't feel like doing the dishes or going to an acquaintance's seventies' themed birthday party (yes, oddly specific, I know) then just say no. No guilt!

Coping with morning sickness

As you read in Rebekah's story, sometimes nothing helps severe morning sickness. But for those of us who experience 'normal' morning sickness, here are some ideas that may provide relief.

- Eat before you get out of bed. As you can gather from its name, morning sickness tends to be worse in the morning, though not always. Eating before getting out of bed can help ease the nausea, so consider keeping a box of dry crackers or nuts on your bedside table.
- Drink throughout the day. Small sips, often, to keep you hydrated, hopefully without vomiting it all up, as can happen if you drink a lot at once.
- Rest and relax. Tiredness and stress can make morning sickness worse, so try to get enough sleep, and relax whenever you can. Prioritise your rest!
- Eat cold meals. If, like me, you feel sick at the smell of pretty much anything cooking, then you will promptly lose your appetite at mealtimes. Eating cold meals, even just a fruit salad, smoothie, sandwich or yoghurt, helped me to at least get something healthy besides dry crackers into my body.
- Just add lemon, ginger and peppermint. Lemon in water, lemon and ginger or peppermint in tea, lemon or peppermint to smell—these foods tend to ease nausea and indigestion, so have them on hand, always.
- Remember, this too shall pass. Morning sickness is an unfortunate reality that pregnant women must endure for an outcome that is so worth it—meeting your baby. Sometimes, when nothing is working and you feel like all you want to do is curl up and cry, take some deep breaths, and tell yourself, this feels bad, really, really bad, but it will be over soon(-ish).

Reflection

Now it's your turn. Have your journal handy so you can use it to answer the questions below. Be as honest as you can be—it's for your eyes only.

- When are you thinking of telling people about your pregnancy? Is there anyone you would like to tell earlier, for an added layer of support, either for the morning sickness period, to talk to about your fears, or in the event of a miscarriage?
- How can your current support system—perhaps your partner or your family—support you right now?
- How can you simplify your life to take time out for nourishment and rest? What are the barriers to this? How can you address these?

2

On Birth: When things don't go as planned

My son was born when I was 35 weeks pregnant—a bit premature but not terribly. It still feels surreal, due to the suddenness of it. I had two weeks left at work before my maternity leave started, so I had to send my boss a text message: 'had the baby this a.m., can't work tomorrow, k thnx bye, cu in 4 months!' (Or something more professional, let's just say.) I hadn't cleaned out my office for my replacement, and I have a sneaking suspicion I might have left a half-filled teacup on my desk, although everyone has been nice enough not to mention it. (Thanks, guys.)

What happened with my son's arrival was this. I went to bed one night. I got up to go to the toilet around an hour later and my water broke. I ~~rushed downstairs in a panic~~ very calmly walked downstairs and told my husband, 'Something weird has just happened'. We called the hospital, and they asked me to come in. Eight hours, a lot of pain, screaming, some gas and air, and an episiotomy later, we had a son.

My experience was relatively straightforward, as far as births go. My sister, on the other hand, recently gave birth in the car—*while they were still driving!* Everyone was okay, though I can't say the same for their car's upholstery.

Lots of women have straightforward experiences, and some don't, as pregnancy and birth stories can be difficult, scary and even dangerous.

Birth trauma

There are few times in life when we find ourselves more vulnerable than during pregnancy. We are sharing our body with another human being, who is completely dependent on us. Our bodies are not fully under our control. For months, we find ourselves sick, sore and tired. Most of us are happy to go through it, knowing that the end result will be worth it. (It is, by the way!)

Then along comes the almost unimaginable reality of birthing a baby. A being that is much too large emerges from a space that is far too small. It's the stuff of science fiction. It is an often long, often very painful process that most of us happily endure (well, happily might be an exaggeration) as a means to an end: bringing our babies earth-side.

What happens when a woman undergoes a traumatic birth? What if her or her baby's life is at risk? Or in other cases if it wasn't, but the woman *felt* like it was?

In a recent Australian study it was found that nearly a third (29 per cent) of Australian mums felt threatened at some point during childbirth.[2] Perhaps this was because of the need for an emergency caesarean, the need for an episiotomy or the use of forceps, an unsupportive hospital staff or partner, or a history of mental health issues. Many of these women said they felt extremely anxious, helpless and even horrified during their birth experience.

In many cultures birth is recognised as a dangerous experience, and full celebrations do not occur until the mum and baby have been fully checked out and deemed to be safe and well. In Western societies the dangers are not considered as much by society in general, given our access to safe medical care. However, it appears it is something that needs to be addressed all over the world given the prevalence of the issue. Not only is this what the research indicates, it is also what I have learned through having frank discussions with many mums.

A psychological injury due to a traumatic birth story—or even perceived trauma during birth—is not uncommon, and trauma or perceived trauma as part of the birth experience can affect a woman's postpartum mental health. Postpartum anxiety, postpartum depression and even post-traumatic stress disorder (PTSD) are all examples of mental health issues that can result. Actual PTSD rates after giving birth are quite low, but women who don't meet all the criteria of PTSD may develop symptoms of the disorder known as 'subsyndromal' PTSD, and reported rates of this are up to a third of postpartum women.[3]

This statistic is massive, and unacceptable, and I strongly feel it warrants further attention and investigation. I also think it is important for women to have realistic expectations of what pregnancy and birth may be like across various scenarios. It would be helpful if our prenatal education included more information on potentially life-saving interventions, such as caesareans, episiotomies and the neonatal intensive care unit (NICU), so that if we do require them we are more aware of what's going on. This is likely to reduce postpartum mental health issues and overall make the whole process less shocking.

Symptoms women may experience after a traumatic or perceived traumatic birth include:

- intrusive thoughts and memories, causing fear and affecting everyday functioning (sleep, social life, mothering, ability to work or study)
- avoidance of sex or personal medical care that reminds them of giving birth, or even of having another child down the track, for fear of repeating the same traumatic experience
- increased levels of anxiety and rumination—anxious about their own or their baby's health, or even possible death
- becoming socially isolated
- struggling with lactation and/or breastfeeding
- problems with relationships.

Her story: Alexis

Alexis underwent a procedure called a 'stretch and sweep'— carried out by a doctor or midwife to attempt to gently initiate labour—because she was a week overdue. Later that day, she began to feel cramping and pain, which worsened to the point where she could not get to sleep that night. She called the hospital and was advised to come in, as it sounded like she might be in labour.

At the hospital she was asked to sit in the waiting room for a long time, and it seemed to her as though the hospital was really crowded. She was greeted by a midwife, who seemed very busy and somewhat harried, and Alexis did not find her to be reassuring or warm at all. The midwife told Alexis she was not in labour and that she should go home. Alexis did not want to leave, but did, only to find the pain worsening. She returned to hospital within a few hours and felt like the staff were 'rolling their eyes' at her, as an anxious, first-time mum.

The pain continued for 48 hours, at the end of which Alexis was still found to be only 1 centimetre dilated. She did not feel supported by hospital staff during this time, and reported feeling alone and scared throughout her labour. After a long two days, the staff became worried about her and the baby's health, and Alexis was suddenly taken into theatre for an emergency caesarean. She did not feel like she had been properly informed about what was happening and had not done any research on what a caesarean involved. She felt rushed and panicked.

After the procedure she was told that she had had some major complications. She did not see her daughter for what felt like a long time after she woke up, and she said she was lying alone in the room, seeing a lot of blood, and not knowing where anyone was. She didn't even know whether her baby was okay.

When she did meet her daughter, someone else had already dressed her, and not in the outfit that Alexis had chosen as her 'first outfit'. Looking back, Alexis recognised that the first outfit she wore would not matter to her daughter and was a 'small thing' but, for some reason, she couldn't get the image of her baby in the wrong outfit, with the other one packed away, getting wrinkled in her bag, out of her mind. She also found it hard to talk to anyone about her feelings, as she worried that they would think she was ungrateful, as everything had turned out okay.

She found it difficult to sleep due to her ruminations about the birth keeping her mind spinning at all hours. She would eventually drift off, only to be awoken by her daughter soon after, and she caught herself resenting her daughter for that. She felt angry at her daughter a lot, and they were not bonding in the way Alexis had envisioned. It was hard to stay 'in the moment' when she was with other people and she began withdrawing and isolating herself. She didn't want to be around anyone, including her daughter. Her relationships with her partner and her friends started to suffer. Alexis felt miserable in the first days and weeks after giving birth.

Her story: Jane

Jane had always been an anxious person. Since she was little she had had major anxiety about getting sick or vomiting. She had never broken any bones, or hurt herself in any real way, but she spent a lot of time worrying that she would. When Jane felt her first contraction she could not believe the amount of pain she was in. Repeatedly, she told her midwife, 'I can't do this!' Her midwife laughed gently, and told her, 'You have no idea how often

I have heard that, but guess what? Then they do it, and so can you.' This helped a bit, but with each contraction Jane felt more and more worried that she would 'break in half'.

Everyone had told her the pain would gradually get worse, and she had heard some women say they were in labour for a whole 24 hours! Jane kept thinking that if she was in this much pain now, after only an hour or two of labour, how much worse would it get?

Eventually, after ten hours of labour it was time to push. The pain hadn't gotten that much worse than it had been in the first hour for Jane, and she had been able to manage her pain and anxiety using the gas and air, but now she felt more anxious about the amount of pain she was in, and worried that she wouldn't be able to do what she needed to do to birth her baby.

The midwives and her husband were telling her to 'Push! Push! I need you to push harder, Jane!' and she began to panic. She felt her chest tightening, and she started to have trouble breathing. Her eyes filled with tears, and she felt like an utter failure as the doctor was called in to do an episiotomy and pull her baby out with forceps, because his heart rate was dropping. She hadn't been able to keep pushing. She felt as though everyone in the room was silently asking her, 'Why couldn't you just push through the pain for the sake of your baby's life, for goodness sake?' She still thinks her husband is wordlessly asking her that.

Jane recovered from the episiotomy, and her baby was just fine, but she still gets short of breath when she is asked if she wants any more kids. She hasn't spoken to her husband about it yet, but she doesn't think she can go through it again.

Let's get practical

These ideas might help you prepare for the process of giving birth, or help you to recover if you do find yourself experiencing any distress following the birth of your baby. It's an extremely sensitive, personal area that can be difficult to process.

Get educated

As we've discussed, having realistic expectations has been shown to ease the transition into an event or life change. Birthing a baby is one of the most major life events you will face. Most hospitals and communities offer a prenatal class to help you prepare for labour and birth. This might take place over the course of a full day, two half-days, or a series of shorter, weekly sessions. Attend this class! Ask lots of questions—about anything you are unsure of. Write down questions you would like to know the answers to, so you don't forget them when it comes time to ask, and write down the answers so you can review them. If anything isn't covered in the class, or you still aren't sure about something, there are a lot of resources on pregnancy and birth online, and there are heaps of books available on this topic. Having up-to-date information will allow you to make a birth plan.

Birth plans

I wish I had prepared mentally for birth, asked more questions, and listened to my midwife's advice to make a birth plan. I think it would have alleviated my anxiety around the unknown and allowed me to make more informed choices around the birthing process. If you have an idea about what you do and don't want to happen during the birth, then you will be less likely to be taken by surprise, or to have an outcome that, in hindsight, you aren't happy with.

Some things you might include in your plan are:

- What, if any, pain relief do you want to use? Some women write that they prefer not to have an epidural, but they want to reserve the right to change their mind on the day. Some women write that they prefer to be asked three times, to make sure they're really sure, before having pain relief administered. Some women write, 'Give me all the drugs!!!'
- Who is allowed in the room? This helps the hospital staff to be your gatekeepers, without putting you in any awkward situations on the day.
- How do you want to labour? Include things like preferred labouring positions, use of the shower or bath, equipment needed.
- Do you want anything special in the room? A photographer, perhaps, or a playlist of relaxation music?
- Include whether you would prefer not to have an episiotomy where possible, preferring to tear naturally.

These are only a few ideas that you could include in your plan. You may feel strongly about some aspects of birth but prefer to leave the rest up to the professionals. You can put in anything you want, as weird and wonderful as it may be!

It may be better to think of birth plans as 'birth wishes' rather than plans though, because as we can see from the women's stories here, things do not always go according to plan. It's important to make informed decisions about our bodies and healthcare during pregnancy and birth. But it is also important to hold these wishes loosely and to be flexible. Be prepared for the fact that things could change. Sometimes the doctors and midwives must make quick calls on treatment, pain relief or surgery. Sometimes circumstances at the hospital don't allow us to get what we want; for example, a bath may be unavailable for a water birth.

Consider your mental health history

When you are planning for birth, it is important to consider your personal and mental health history, and to make your healthcare team aware of this as well. If you have any history of trauma, anxiety or panic, you may find the process of birth triggers your anxiety. The significance of the event, the intense setting, the pain, the unknown, and the heightened emotions all together can be overwhelming for anyone, but even more so for someone with a history of mental health issues or a trauma background. If your healthcare team is aware, then they are more likely to be able to help you with a personalised approach to the birth.

It's important to plan mentally and emotionally prior to the birth. If you haven't already, you may like to speak to a doctor, who can refer you to an appropriate psychologist or other mental health professional to speak to about personalised strategies for managing your anxiety while giving birth. Things like deep breathing, grounding or relaxation techniques, while they seem simple, can be invaluable in managing both the physiological and mental symptoms of anxiety. (These strategies will be discussed further in Chapter 9, 'On Postpartum Anxiety'.)

Gather support

Research has shown more positive psychological outcomes post-partum for women who have a good supportive social network. If possible, have a support person attend your prenatal appointments and, more importantly, the birth with you. In most cases, this will be a woman's romantic partner. If you are a single mum, or your partner is not available to attend, consider taking a person you trust, whether that is a friend or a family member who has shown themself to be supportive to you in the past. In addition, having a solid social support network in the early days and weeks postpartum is also important. Consider inviting people to come over and meet baby, accept help and support where offered, and try not to isolate yourself following the birth.

Postpartum distress

If you have already given birth and it did not go to plan, for whatever reason, firstly, I'm sorry. It is an incredibly personal and important life experience, and if it caused you distress and trauma, this can mean a grieving process for what you had hoped for. Please allow yourself to do this in your own way. It is important that your own feelings around this are validated by others, but also by yourself. You don't need to forget all about it because 'everything turned out okay'.

Talking about your distress is helpful. Many women find it incredibly cathartic just to talk about their birth experience with another person. If you are not ready to do this with a person you know in real life, there are some great internet forums for people who have experienced birth trauma that you can check out. Many women find it especially important to talk to their partner about how they are feeling. Partners are not mind readers, unfortunately, and letting them know how you are going and why you may be acting in certain ways may help prevent arguments, misunderstandings and subsequently feelings of being even more alone. Knowing where you are at emotionally may also let your partner know that you need some extra support, quality time, time off, or help with certain things.

Self-care

Take care of yourself. As well as the fact that you are important—because *you just are*—some women struggle to take that on board and need an extra incentive to look after themselves, so here goes: you are your baby's most important asset! It is the opposite of selfish to place yourself in a place of high importance right now; it is vital for your baby's well-being. You are everything they have.

Here's a tried-and-true metaphor to illustrate what I mean. Think of it like being on an aeroplane, when the flight attendant says in the safety talk at the start of the flight, you need to fit your own oxygen mask before helping babies and children with theirs.

You are going to be no good to anyone if you are not taken care of first. As they say, you can't pour from an empty cup. So, allow yourself time to heal, look after yourself and let your partner, family or friends take over your usual responsibilities where you can, so you have space to do so.

Reflection

Now it's your turn! Grab your journal, make a fresh cup of tea or coffee, and let's think about you for a few minutes. Write as much or as little as you wish—this is just for you.

- What are your hopes, dreams and goals for your pregnancy and birthing experience? (Remember to hold these in mind, but loosely, in case things don't work out the way you wish.)
- What fears do you have regarding your pregnancy and birth? Have you spoken to anyone about them?
- What questions do you have for your midwives or doctor next time you see them?
- What are you most looking forward to about meeting your baby for the first time?
- What is the one thing that your partner, or support person, could do that would be most helpful to you in this stage of your pregnancy, at the birth or in parenthood? Have you told them?
- If you have already had your baby, how was your experience? Do you have unresolved feelings around the experience, and would it help to talk about them?

3

On Taking Baby Home:
A steep learning curve

When my son was born prematurely, I assumed we would be in the hospital for a while. Fortunately, though, he didn't have any significant health issues and he didn't require any time in the neonatal intensive care unit (NICU), so we were good to go. What I was not prepared for was being in hospital for *only one night*. Due to a severe, almost biblical 'no room at the inn' situation, the maternity ward was full to the brim. Mind you, I was also happy to be discharged.

I was sharing a room with four other women and their babies. It was *loud*. At least one baby was always wailing. None of us slept. My roomies and I all shuffled around with our little plastic see-through tubs on wheels containing our new offspring, wordlessly acknowledging each other with glassy, vacant eyes and silent nods of solidarity. I never spoke to anyone. I think we were all in shock. What just happened? Are my insides still inside me?

Just as I wasn't prepared for such a short hospital stay, I was also not prepared for the fact that, when it was time to leave, the hospital *just let us go.* No exam or pop quiz. No licence. No last-minute pep talks or words of advice. No marching band leading us down the hallway towards the car. (Okay, this last one might have been a stretch.) At one point when we were leaving, a lady chased us down the hallway and I thought 'well, finally . . .' But it turned out she was just returning a wool beanie we had dropped. (I don't know why, but I had bought about a million of them in the hospital. What did I think I was going to do with them all in the middle of a Queensland summer?)

We left, and I remember thinking, 'Do these people know that I have no idea what I'm doing?' I'd had more extensive training for my first job at KFC than for this. My training for being a mum was one (optional) day at the local community centre on birthing a baby—and nothing but *nothing* on what happens after you take the baby home. Though there are community mothers' groups that can help with this, they don't start until later, *after* the baby arrives. For me, it was eight weeks after I'd had my son, due to him being born close to Christmas and everything shuts down over that period.

Because we thought we still had more than a month to go before his birth, we were not prepared for our son's arrival—not just mentally, but in every sense of the word. Our bassinet was on back order. We hadn't fitted the car seat. We had no baby monitor. Our house hadn't been vacuumed in longer than I want to admit to (hey, I was pregnant okay), and it was a dog hair-infested war zone.

'What if he's allergic to dogs?' I suddenly panicked while still in hospital, thinking about the state of our home.

'I hope he likes sleeping outside', my husband replied, referring to the baby, of course, not the dog—joking of course, but still earning an eye-roll from me.

So the day I spent in hospital, learning to feed, burp and change the baby, my husband chased up the bassinet, bought nappies, fitted the car seat, and vacuumed and cleaned the house. And that was it! We were parents and, from here on out, we were on our own. Now what?

Now, you start learning. Learning so, so much, every day. It's extremely taxing, learning critical, life-sustaining skills under the most unaccommodating of circumstances: sleep deprivation, hormonal changes and stress. These make learning important new things an uphill battle, but learning happens, nonetheless.

Your brain is amazing! In these first weeks, you will learn about your baby (complex creatures that they are), about baby *stuff* (also freaking complex!) and about yourself as a parent (mind-blowingly complex!). There are so many things to know and learn as a new mum that it can be overwhelming.

Getting to know your baby

You've probably heard that all babies do is cry, eat, sleep and poop. That is true actually, but what you wouldn't expect is that each of those things is a veritable minefield to figure out. Honestly, I don't know how previous generations parented without Google. I guess they read real paper books and called or visited one another in the flesh. How odd.

If you are like me, and most of the mums I chatted to, you will spend the first few weeks of motherhood getting to know your baby's 'signs'. Each baby has their own special signals to let you know what they need, which are very handy. It's extremely cool that babies can communicate with us right from the beginning! Lots of babies show similar signs, so both Google and other parents can likely provide some good answers for what the heck your baby is doing now. Some of their signs are so funny. Some examples of my son's were: sucking on his hands when he was hungry, pulling his ears or making jerky robot moves when he was tired, lifting his legs up in the air when he was gassy, and crying when he was . . . well, pretty much everything actually. That bit wasn't funny.

If you are like me, you will use the time you don't spend staring at your baby trying to decipher their signs on your phone or laptop typing in increasingly specific questions and hoping that other babies out there are just as weird as yours. Guess what? They are! Babies are just weird in general!

Mothers' groups

Mothers' groups can be such a wealth of information and support when you are a new mum. In Australia, when you give birth for the first time, you are placed into a community mothers' group. Basically, this entails weekly meetings with a smallish group of other mums and a community midwife, who facilitates the meeting. There is often a guest speaker who talks about their area of expertise. We had a dentist, a lactation consultant, and a swim instructor speak at ours. (The swim instructor spoke about safe bathing, *not* training for the 100-metre freestyle, in case you were wondering.) On weeks when there wasn't a guest speaker, the community midwife spoke about general topics, like feeding and sleeping.

I loved my group, which was a stroke of luck considering that you don't necessarily have much in common with the group you're placed in, other than you live in the same general postcode and are likely to have engaged in amorous activities at around the same time nine months earlier. My group was down-to-earth, casual, real and funny. I have heard other women say that their group was a nightmare, usually due to feeling judged or mums competing with each other. We didn't have any of that, thank goodness. It all depends on the mums you are placed with, I guess. There is no requirement to keep going if you don't find it helpful, or if it is a source of stress for you. If you hate it, stop going. No worries.

When I say we weren't competing, I mean, we weren't judging or one-upping each other, but we probably *were* all secretly comparing, trying to figure out if we were 'normal'. Mothers' group, at least in the first weeks, was a desperate ploy for validation disguised as chit-chat. It was an attempt to seem nonchalant while you secretly sussed out what all the other babies were doing, firing off as many questions as you could within the relatively short space of time before the tea and bickies appeared (and before the

Kingstons and Monte Carlos disappeared). Meanwhile, others attempted to do the same to you. Questions rocketed back and forth like tennis balls, one streaming into the next until no one appeared casual anymore.

We all probably appeared slightly frenzied for the first few weeks. But we were in it together, and once a week, for that two-hour period, my world expanded. I was part of something, and I was with people who totally got where I was at. I recommend people at least give a mothers' group a shot. If you hate it, no harm done, just don't go back. If you love it, there are lots of benefits.

Baby routines

You might have heard the words 'baby routine' bandied about. Babies are creatures of habit and thrive on routine. However, the first weeks of your baby's life are not the best time to try and implement strict schedules. Even full-term babies are too immature to fit into any kind of feeding or sleeping schedule when they are first born, so trying to establish a strict, scheduled, time-based routine right away is an exercise in futility and frustration. It won't work. Your baby won't do what you think they *should* be doing, *when* you think they should be doing it. They won't do what the books say, and you will drive yourself batty trying to make it happen. Now is the time to recover from birth, get to know your baby, and just be.

As the baby gets a bit older, there will be time to establish schedules and routines, and this will be a very good thing. There are heaps of excellent resources out there that can teach you how to implement these. It's a matter of finding one that sits right with you, and suits you, your baby and your family's life.

There are certain things that do need to happen as part of your baby's day from the very beginning, though, specifically, sleeping, eating and 'playing'. I put playing in quotation marks because depending on bub's age, playing may just involve her lying on the floor and staring at a shadow on the wall, or staring at your face. Your face will be fascinating to your baby.

As they get older, playing may involve singing songs, reading stories or peekaboo. There is no need for lots of expensive toys to motivate your baby; they are plenty stimulated just watching you and their surroundings. Everything is brand new = everything is stimulating! They are learning the world from scratch.

It is important to place your baby on their tummy and on their back frequently throughout the day, to help with their strength, coordination and overall development. This will also allow your baby to see the world from different angles and keep them endlessly entertained.

There are important things to include in your baby's day, but now is not the time to structure them into a strict, timed schedule. You need to respond to your baby's cues and signs and allow *them* to show *you* what timings will work for them regarding these activities. You should have some idea about how many naps and feeds a baby generally needs in a day, and how long they can stay awake for as a guide, but your timings should be flexible. There is no point stressing about keeping your baby awake so they can have a play because that book said they should, when they are clearly tired and need a sleep. There is no point spending a frustrating hour trying to settle a very awake baby, who will tire themselves out naturally with just a bit of extra playtime on the floor. Allowing your baby to develop their own feeding, sleeping and playing routine at the beginning will take a load of stress off you, and generally make things more peaceful for the whole family.

You can set the groundwork for later routines from the beginning, though. As you get to know your baby's cues and signs, respond to them in a consistent manner, and your baby will take comfort in learning what's coming next. If your baby is rubbing his fists in his eyes, and this is his 'tired sign', then pop him into bed with a lullaby. In turn, he will learn to associate a lullaby with sleep. When you are ready to set up a more structured sleep routine in a few months—if he hasn't fallen into his own—he will already associate lullabies with bedtime, and you will have an easier time putting him down to sleep. When you sing, he will be able to anticipate what's coming next: sleep. This is the beginning of a baby-led routine.

The first weeks are for rest, recovery, and learning about your baby—and then responding to their needs in a consistent, predictable and gentle manner. You do need to include certain things in their day—sleeping, feeding, playing—but leave it to baby to determine the timings of these for now. You will probably find that your baby will fall into their own routine, and this will help your life to feel somewhat predictable again. But try to let them show you their routine for now, rather than the other way around. If a routine doesn't establish itself with time, and your baby is getting older, *then* look at resources to help you establish a routine. Until then, let baby take the lead. It's one less thing on your plate!

Baby 'stuff'

I was gobsmacked by the amount of random stuff I had to learn after giving birth. As if making a human wasn't hard enough, now I apparently needed a degree in engineering just to figure out how to cart him around by car, pram or carrier. As silly as it sounds, I was proud of myself for learning so much new stuff. As a notoriously 'spatially challenged' person who has yet to figure out how to open a new cling wrap box without destroying it, there were some aspects of new motherhood that rendered me completely discombobulated!

It took me two weeks before I felt confident with the baby capsule and how to put my son in the car. The breast pump was a force to be reckoned with, and I felt like I was working for NASA when I tried to fit the pram into the boot of the car. There was the cloth nappy and swaddle cloth origami, the baby carrier perplexity, the bath equipment bewilderment and the flat packs sent from Hades (aka IKEA). But I muddled through.

My biggest tips: ask for help if you need it, as many times as you need to; practise with the pram, baby wrap and capsule a few times before venturing out of the house, so as not to get stuck in the carpark; and, most of all, give yourself a break. It's a steep learning curve, lots of new stuff to learn, and you're doing great.

Plus, you just made a human—you can be forgiven if it takes you a while to learn their various accoutrements.

Words of wisdom

I asked a bunch of mums for some words of wisdom that they wished they could go back in time and tell their new-mum selves, in the hope that future new mums would benefit from their collective, seasoned wisdom. I heard these gems.

- No one is going to give you a gold medal for doing it all, and you don't have to be 'the best' at this—there's no competition except in your own mind.
- It's just a phase, it's just a phase, it's just a phase.
- The time goes by so fast, so take more videos and photos, and be in them with baby, not just behind the camera.
- Only use parenting books as a guide—what works for others may not work for you and things may not pan out the way the books say they should because your baby hasn't read them.
- Relax, she's not yet mobile—you have time to shave your legs *and* wash your hair in the shower . . . she's not going anywhere.
- Recognise the symptoms of postpartum anxiety and depression—if I'd known what was happening, I would have gotten help sooner.
- It is okay to supplement with formula or even stop breast-feeding altogether—your health matters too, and formula is awesome.
- You are enough—really you are . . . more than, even.

- Nobody else knows what they are doing either, so don't worry so much.
- Your baby is going to love you so much!
- Your heart is now walking around outside your body. The love is awesome but can also be scary as all hell. The thought of losing it can send you into a vulnerable panic.
- This too shall pass.

Her story: Kirsten

Kirsten and her partner had only been together for fourteen months when Kirsten took a pregnancy test. Her heart froze when she saw the double pink lines.

'What have we done?' she thought. She said she could count on three fingers how many times they had been intimate in the past four months, and she had always had it in her mind that she would have trouble conceiving—she didn't know why. This news was a shock, to say the least.

Kirsten developed severe pain and fatigue that forced her to leave her job as a nurse at 16 weeks pregnant, for safety reasons as well as the pain—she was dealing with very unwell patients and did not feel safe in that job while pregnant. This meant she did not qualify for any government maternity leave. She did not feel bonded with baby during pregnancy but figured (and hoped) that would come after birth. Though she and her partner bought all the baby furniture and attended all the necessary scans and appointments, she thinks they were in denial that having a baby was going to be a life-changing event.

When her son was born Kirstin felt . . . well, nothing. She thought this might have been shock. But once she got home from hospital she still didn't feel that 'overwhelming feeling of love' that people talk about. What she did feel was regret. They were the first of their friends to have a baby, and so they didn't really feel they had much support or understanding from their friends, just because those friends hadn't been in their shoes yet.

Kirsten said that her mind was on a 24/7 loop of 'what have we done?' She considered adoption but didn't think she could ever really do that. She considered suicide.

She knew what she was feeling was common, but not normal. She told the midwives, who set her up with some extra home visits. She saw a psychologist who reinforced what she knew: these feelings were common but not normal. The psychologist said the feelings would probably pass in the next six weeks.

Kirsten found that having this timeline really helped her to cope—there was light at the end of the tunnel. Although it took her a long time to bond with her son, the initial regret she felt when he was born passed within a few months. Kristen is pleased to say, she now couldn't live without him—he brings her so much joy and happiness. He is soon going to be a big brother!

Let's get practical

Here are some strategies that might help you as you navigate your way through the early days of motherhood.

Don't seek perfection

Having a new baby at home gives us a free pass to toss perfectionism out the window. Though we should never feel we have to be perfect, lots of us, me included, often feel like we do. We feel embarrassed if someone drops by the house and the dishes aren't done, and the floors aren't clean. We hesitate to answer the door if we have no make-up on and we are wearing the same stained tracksuit for the third day in a row.

When you have a new baby, it's not possible to keep on top of this stuff—at least that's what I found out, because I sure didn't! The people that make the effort to drop in to visit you and your baby do not care about the state of your laundry pile—if they do, then their opinion is not worth worrying about. They are there to see you and your baby, not your house.

It might not be love at first sight

Just like every other important type of relationship in life, mums and babies get to know each other and form connections in different ways. Sometimes it is love at first sight, an instant connection, the stuff Hollywood movies are made of. Sometimes relationships develop over time, as you slowly get to know one another. For me, with my son, it was the latter. Bonding took time. It was this way for many of the other mums I chatted to as well. Many of us felt guilty about this. There is a myth in society that we will immediately get that 'maternal instinct' and feel love at first sight with our babies. It does happen for some people, but not always. It's okay if it takes some time. There is no need to rush your relationship. You have your whole lives together!

Don't stew the small stuff

One of the most important lessons I learned when I was a new mum was to not stew the small stuff. There are enough big, new, scary and important things to focus on, without spending the whole time analysing every small, perceived threat or offence. That might be your partner saying something insensitive without thinking, or a stranger saying something rude to you in the shops. I tended to stew on this type of stuff for way longer than was necessary when I was a new mum. A friend suggested we may do this because it is more comfortable to think about the 'little' insignificant things in life than to 'go there' with the big, important stuff. We often spend our precious time thinking about the small stuff to avoid thinking about the major life issues, the stuff that actually does require our time and energy. For example, we probably don't need to still be dwelling on the funny look we got from the lady in the supermarket when our baby was screaming the place down, an hour after we arrived home. I spent (wasted) too much time thinking about inconsequential negative moments as a new mum, and it was exhausting! I bet I'm not alone in that.

Don't resist change—roll with it

I spent a good part of my son's infancy resisting change. I subconsciously pushed back against the changes that having a newborn necessitated. I couldn't get used to the lack of autonomy—of never being alone or sleeping or eating whenever I wanted. I wish, looking back, that I had been prepared for the psychological adjustment to becoming a mum. I wish I had known that having these emotions was normal and to be expected. I wish I had known that, because then I think I could have accepted it.

Rather than push back against the season I was in or trying to hurry through it, I could have embraced it with a 'this too shall pass' mentality, and even enjoyed it as a passing season. There are a lot of positives to the newborn season that I rushed through in my hurry to outrun the adjustment, rather than just live in the moment. I put conditions on my own happiness. I thought I would be okay, but only once my son slept through the night, or when he ate solid foods, or when he could sit up by himself. Learning the art of contentment, of being content right where you are at now, is crucial as a new parent.

There is a powerful quote by Eckhart Tolle that reflects what I mean perfectly:

Always say 'yes' to the present moment. What could be more futile, more insane, than to create inner resistance to what already is? What could be more insane than to oppose life itself, which is now and always now? Surrender to what is. Say 'yes' to life—and see how life suddenly starts working for you rather than against you.

Don't lose yourself

When I was a new mum, I lost myself a bit. My identity became mum and not much else for a while. I was so overwhelmed with keeping my head above water that I felt like I needed all my mental and physical energy just to keep treading water. Survival mode is fine for a short burst of time, but it's not sustainable. We need to remember our own identity outside of parenting. Our identity as a person, not just a mum, and living according to our personal values, is important. It is freeing to find something that's just for you to focus on outside of motherhood from the very beginning. (Identity will be discussed more in Chapter 12.)

For me, when my son was a few months old I suddenly had the wake-up call that I was still a whole entire person outside of being his mum. I remembered that writing and storytelling were a vital part of my soul, and once I started writing again, journaling, blogging and writing articles and stories, I found a part of me that I'd almost forgotten existed. Start as you mean to go on. This could be a creative outlet, your own health and fitness goals, your spiritual journey, social justice endeavours or your social life. Make sure you remember what it is that makes you you, and revel in it.

One primary adviser

I strongly suggest having in your life one central person you can trust for baby-related advice. This person may be your doctor, midwife or paediatrician. They should be someone professional who knows what they are talking about, and also someone who is easily accessible and approachable so that you feel heard and supported. Choose to listen to them, and only them, and ignore all the other baby advice, unless it aligns with theirs.

If you listen to every Tom, Dick and Harry out there, you will end up with a million differing opinions on *everything* and become completely bamboozled. As a new mum I would often talk to my GP, then the maternal child health nurse, then the lactation consultant, then my GP again, and none of their advice was the same! I was so confused until I decided to stick with one primary person as my baby guru. I chose my GP, because he was nice, non-judgemental, close to home, accessible *and* he bulk-billed—always a plus!

Social media—pros and cons

Social media use in new motherhood is a tricky area. Part of me says ban it! Ban it all! It can lead to comparisons, feelings of failure, and loneliness and the fear of missing out that is so common during new parenthood. Seeing other parents' seemingly perfect lives makes us wonder how they have it all together. You can never measure up to an Instagram photo—that isn't real life.

Newborn parenting is a tough gig. It's easy to make something look good on social media. People aren't generally deceptive, just excited and proud. But what you see on social media are other people's highlight reels, a filter on their home lives. It makes our own real lives feel like blooper reels. No wonder when we compare ourselves to them we come up short. Never mind that we also just posted our own perfectly filtered photo, shot during the two minutes between baby cries. We know that our posts are not a reflection of our real lives, yet we think other peoples' are.

We also see people out socialising via social media. They look to be having a great time without us, and we can feel like our life has ended because we are at home with the baby. We feel left out. This can lead to a sense of loneliness and isolation.

Social media can make us feel 'less-than'.

However . . . social media was also a huge form of social connectivity and support for me as a new mum, especially as one who didn't have any family nearby. It allowed my family to see photos and updates on our lives every day. Some weeks, it was the only way I communicated with anyone outside of my immediate family. As an introvert, I didn't mind that—it was a good balance of still feeling like I was part of the world, without having to venture out into it before I was ready or able. In addition to my 'actual real-life friends' I also found a hugely supportive group of mums online on social media, and to this day, though I haven't met many of them, we remain friends who talk daily, and support each other through the different ages and stages of parenthood.

I'm inclined to say with regards to social media: do what feels right for you. If it is causing you any distress, if it's making you feel left out of things, or making you sad, then you may want to limit it. If you find you are comparing yourself to other people's online presence, step away! But, if you're not negatively affected by it and you enjoy using it, then feel free to scroll away happily.

If you choose to limit social media, rather than eliminate it, an effective method can be to simply delete the applications off your phone. People find that if they need to log on to their computer to access social media, they are less likely to use it out of automatic habit, and to only use it when they have a specific purpose.

Enlist support

Babies interpret love as someone being there and responding to their immediate needs in a gentle way. They don't read our minds or know if we don't feel head over heels in love with them right away. If we struggle with the newborn stage, it is a relief to know that the long-term attachment and love of our baby are not dependent on how we feel in those early weeks. We must find ways to safely and gently meet the immediate needs of our babies (feeding, settling to sleep and changing them), despite how we feel. This might mean enlisting a support system to help with both the baby's needs and your own.

Accept practical support when offered—every time! Give people specific jobs. In Kirsten's story, her friends would have been more than willing to help; they just didn't know how. Ask for what you need. An example might be to ask your friends for meals to freeze for when you need a break from cooking, or to ask your partner to take over baby duty while you take a bath.

It is also important to seek emotional support. As Kirsten discovered, overwhelming feelings are common in the early weeks of motherhood. That doesn't mean they are normal or that we should just put up with them. We must seek the support of our partners, friends and family. There are also professionals whose job it is to listen and give you practical strategies on how to adjust to your new job as mum.

Your first point of contact may be your local GP, the hospital you gave birth at, or your maternal child health nurse. They may refer you to a counsellor, social worker or psychologist. If you don't feel comfortable with the first person you see, please don't give up. Like with any relationship, it can take some time to 'click' with someone. If you feel like you are unlikely to connect with the person you are seeking help from, there is no shame in trying someone new. As a psychologist, I promise, this is okay—we will not be offended!

'Just be' with your baby

Spend some time getting to know your baby, with the sole purpose being to just *be* with them. Babies love looking at faces—it's one of their favourite pastimes. As you spend pressure-free time with your baby, just being, just looking, your bond will grow. You will fall more and more in love with them, helped along by the flood of 'love chemicals' oxytocin and dopamine. As you hold, rock or feed your baby, a stream of hormones and chemicals will flood through your body, and your baby's body, cementing your bond. You don't have to have given birth for this to happen either. Studies show that both fathers and adoptive parents get hits of oxytocin and dopamine too.[4]

The good news for those among us who did not feel like they bonded with their baby right away is that there is no specific window of opportunity for bonding. My research indicated that for many mums this takes place slowly, over weeks or even months. I get that taking the time to just be with your baby can be tough when stressed, busy and exhausted, so try to take the pressure off and do what you can.

Reflection

Find someone to cover mum duties for you, grab your journal and a fresh cuppa and spend some time reflecting on these questions.

- What do you think it will be like, having a new baby? What are you most looking forward to? Is there anything you are dreading or feeling anxious about?
- Who are your 'people'? Do you have people lined up (even if just in your mind) who you know you can talk to? Someone who might be able to help with practical support? Have a think about the 'support team' you could assemble.
- How are you coping with having a new baby? Is it all you thought it would be? Is there something that is different? Have you met or heard of anyone having a similar experience? How did it feel when you found out that someone shared your experience?
- Did you relate to Kirsten's story, of regretting becoming pregnant or having a baby? Did you feel resentment? How is that going now?
- What are you grateful for today, in this moment? Spend some time reflecting on the things, big and small, that make you feel happy, thankful or hopeful.

- What could you and your baby do together today, to 'just be' together? Maybe consider learning some lullabies to sing to her or reading some stories. Even just spending time lying together on the floor and looking at each other is a beautiful way to bond. What would you like to do together today?
- Who would you most like and trust to be your primary baby adviser?

4

On the Baby Blues: What no one told me about week one

One of the most surprising—and not in a good way—aspects of new motherhood, for me, was the way my body, specifically my hormones, reacted to giving birth. I had heard of the 'baby blues' before, but it was described as 'weepiness' or a general 'blue mood' brought on by lack of sleep or stress. Instead, a sudden, brutal feeling of *hopelessness* and acute depression landed on me. It started on day three postpartum, and the feelings were so intense I remember it like it was yesterday.

No one had warned me about it! I am including it here, in its own special chapter, because I had *no idea* what was happening to me on day three of my son's life. If I can help someone, even one woman, cope with this phenomenon a bit better than I did, I feel that writing about it will have been worth it. As discussed, knowing what to expect is a huge predictor of coping in the postpartum period. This became very apparent to me during week one of my motherhood journey, when I thought there was something seriously wrong with me.

A lot of people think that the first week postpartum is going to be all magic, bonding, snuggles and lullabies. I did. It was an unrealistic perception, and I wonder why we mums don't talk about it much. During week one, I didn't even recognise myself in the woman sobbing on the couch, oblivious to anything good in the world. Who was she, and how was she ever going to be a mum if she couldn't even see past tomorrow?

The uncomfortable reality is that up to 70 per cent of women experience the baby blues in the first week after giving birth.[5] The severity ranges—some women experience a really mild form of the blues, while others are much more significantly impacted. The blues normally rear their ugly head around day three, and last for around a week, usually improving by around day ten (give or take a few days). But none of the women I knew warned me about it. When I spoke to other mums, they were equally as shocked about the way they were feeling during their first postpartum week.

Most women report symptoms like feeling sad, mood swings, insomnia, loss of appetite and anger in the first week after giving birth. If the baby blues are severe, or last longer than a couple of weeks, this can increase the risk of a mum developing postpartum depression. (Postpartum depression is discussed further in Chapter 8.) It is important to note, if you are yet to give birth, that the baby blues is likely to happen to you, and it might present mildly or severely, but it's not an illness. It's a normal, physical, hormonal reaction that will most likely go away by itself without any medical intervention. But it can be *really* difficult while it's happening.

The baby blues turned my whole world on its axis. I had been residing in a sleep-deprived but generally euphoric bubble for two days and then bam! I felt awful for no identifiable reason. Everything felt tragic, hopeless and dark, and I didn't have any idea why. It was so weird. I felt like I was outside of myself, looking in, but not seeing much. It was scary.

For me, the blues were really, really bad for around three days—by 'really bad', I mean, I could not see anything getting better and I regretted ever becoming a mother. I thought I'd ruined my life and my baby's by default. Then one day I woke up feeling a bit better. I gradually improved over the week, and by week two I was okay. I have gone on to experience emotional 'ups and downs' since, but *nothing* as intense or acute as that first week postpartum. Thank goodness.

That week was a huge challenge—dark and bordering on dangerous. If I had known what was coming, I may have been able to lie low and wait it out, knowing that it would pass, but I didn't know. No one talks about it! This meant that I blamed myself: I'm not cut out to be a mum; I'm selfish; I'm *crazy*, and I've made a mistake; I've ruined our lives. On and on it went. My mind was a hamster wheel of negativity. I would swing between being stuck in the past—regretful, remorseful, 'if only' thoughts— and catapulting into the future—worried, anxious and 'what if' thoughts. I was never in the moment. The moment was too hard! I was exhausted.

My introverted temperament was magnified during this time—I elevated to full-on hermit. I didn't want to leave the house. I remember one day, when my husband asked if I wanted to come with him to the chemist, I ran away from him and hid in the bathroom, sobbing! I don't know why. There was no logic going on. Every problem in my life was magnified in my head. Everything I'd previously been slightly concerned about had suddenly escalated to disaster-mode. I looked at everything through a negative lens.

Historically, the cause of the baby blues has been unclear. Scientists thought that it might have been solely due to the adjustment to parenthood—the realities of the loss of autonomy and freedom, and the huge responsibility kicking in. But then why were mothers also reporting the same symptoms after giving birth to their subsequent children? Surely there was more to it than that. They discovered that indeed there was.

Scientists now know that there are neurobiological factors associated with the blues. Namely, there is a rapid drop in oestrogen in the first three days after giving birth, and an increase in the levels of the enzyme monoamine oxidase A (MAO-A). Levels of MAO-A were found to be up to 43 per cent higher in new mums than in child-free women, or mums who had given birth years ago. MAO-A levels in new mums were found to peak on day five, postpartum. This timing is consistent with what happened to me, and what a lot of mums described when I asked them about their first week of motherhood. MAO-A's job is to break down the neurotransmitters serotonin, dopamine and norepinephrine. These neurotransmitters are huge influencers and regulators of our mood. If they aren't correctly balanced, it can cause us to feel sad, angry or anxious, and even to develop more serious mental health disorders down the track.

Again, it is important to note that the baby blues experience is *not* an illness. For most women, the increased levels of MAO-A are temporary and quickly return to normal. This doesn't mean that you shouldn't seek help if you need some support.

Her story: Lara

Lara enjoyed a healthy and happy pregnancy. She loved the feeling of being pregnant and enjoyed attending all her prenatal appointments and check-ups. She loved eating healthily, and exercising, knowing that each time she did, she was improving her own health and the health of her baby. She had never felt better, despite the morning sickness. She had overcome depression in her teen years and had spent her twenties so far committed to healthy living, knowing that this helped her to stave off the symptoms of what she calls her 'black dog'. During her pregnancy journey, the midwives and doctors praised her for the way she was looking after herself, and her baby. They kept a close eye on her, due to her history of depression.

Suddenly, when her daughter was born, Lara felt like all the attention of the midwives and doctors went from her well-being to that of this 'crying, screaming thing in the bassinet'. She felt like no one noticed her, and she was 'just here to make sure the baby was okay'. She felt completely overlooked.

Lara said that she doesn't remember much from the first week postpartum, but she does recall intense feelings. She remembers wanting her mum a lot. She remembers feeling as though her life was over. She remembers feeling as though she was not cut out to be a mum, and like she was going to mess up this baby's life, and her own too.

She cried all the time. Lara did not really know why she was crying, and she began to feel even worse when people would ask her what was wrong. She didn't have an answer, and then she began feeling guilty, because at least she had a healthy baby. So many of her friends had suffered miscarriage and infertility, and she felt guilty that she was *this* upset over 'nothing'.

Her husband tried to help, by trying to figure out what was wrong, but she didn't find it helpful. He would try to console her by talking to her about how it was just her hormones levelling out, and how the upsetting feelings would pass soon. Lara said she knew this logically, but she did not *feel* like they were going to pass. She found his efforts pressuring, for she had no answer for him and she felt he wouldn't let up until he had 'solved her problem'.

Every time the baby cried, Lara cried. She worried that she was doing severe emotional damage to her daughter by crying so much. She wondered if she would ever feel 'normal' again. She grabbed every opportunity she could to be away from her daughter. She had long showers, and then after the water went cold, she sat on the bathroom floor with the water running, so her husband would think she was still in the shower.

Lara tried to minimise the time she spent socialising with the baby. She went to the gym at five days postpartum. As she said,

'I didn't want to do any exercise; I just wanted to feel like the old me.' She feels guilty disclosing this now but wanted to be honest about the way she was feeling.

She had been told that these feelings would pass. After a week she went to her GP, because she was still feeling really low. He reassured her that he would keep a close eye on her, and wanted to see her again the following week, and that it was normal for the blues to last for a week or so. She believed him and went home feeling more positive once she had spoken about her feelings out loud. She had thought they were dreadful, selfish and hateful; but it turned out they were quite normal!

Lara went back to the doctor the next week with good news to report: she felt much better. She described it as though a fog had lifted, and she was able to start enjoying being a new mum. Yes, she still had tough days, but overall she felt more like herself again, and ready to transition into this new phase in her life.

Let's get practical

Some people didn't, or won't, experience the baby blues post-partum, and if that's you, feel free to skip over this part if it's not relevant. If you are feeling the blues, these ideas might help you through that first week postpartum. Remember, though, this advice isn't meant to replace your healthcare team and any strategies you use should be done in conjunction with them.

Tell someone

It sometimes seems as though it is socially unacceptable to be struggling emotionally after giving birth. We are supposed to be happy, right? If not, why not? We feel ungrateful, because our baby is all right and we are lucky—there is nothing 'wrong'. But we feel so bad. Perhaps, then, we should surround ourselves in that first week with people who get it. Now that you know what you may potentially face, you can warn your partner, friends or family members who will be around that you may not be yourself in week one. Tell them how you would like them to assist during the week—hugs, space, a break, company, a shoulder to cry on, a chance to talk, coffee?

Plan to your temperament

Think in advance about how you would like to manage these emotions when or if they arrive. Are you an extrovert who copes with things by having lots of visitors around? Are you an introvert who needs alone time, who should perhaps limit the number of visitors in that first week in case of potentially feeling over-whelmed? Let people know in advance what you need from them, bearing in mind your temperament, so you don't have to deal with awkward moments at an already vulnerable time.

Prepare for self-care

Consider preparing some self-care items for your first week postpartum. We all worry about packing our hospital bags and preparing the baby's nursery, but let's talk about investing in ourselves for a minute. Fill a container with whatever you may need to treat yourself with in that first week, with the expectation that it might be difficult for you emotionally. Some ideas are favourite foods, bath treats for a relaxing bubble bath, books or magazines you will look forward to reading, a journal. Or you could plan to binge on a TV series.

Find your flow

An important form of catharsis and release for me when I was a new mum was writing—still is. I called my first blog 'She Writes to Exhale', because I did! I wrote about my struggles, my wins, my frustrations and pretty much everything. Lots of times I deleted what I wrote. That's okay; it was just for me. Writing may or may not be your type of thing, so think about what is—sport, music, art, reading, meditation. Choose something that gives you a sense of 'flow'. The concept of flow was named by positive psychologist Mihaly Csikszentmihalyi. Flow is when you are 'in the zone'; you are completely engaged and focused on your activity. When you are in your flow, you often lose all sense of time, and feel lots of positive energy. You feel better after completing the activity. It is time-consuming but energising, not draining. What activities have you tried in the past that helped you feel that way? Find a way, with support, to do that!

Note: I originally wrote about the 'Baby Blues' for www.mother.ly.com. You can find the original article on their website.[6]

Reflection

It's your turn again! Grab your journal and think about your first week of parenthood, whether that time is in the future or the past.

- Is there someone who you trust, that you could speak to candidly about their first week of motherhood? What kinds of questions would you love to ask someone having read this chapter? Perhaps you could write down some questions for them to answer, if they feel comfortable doing so.

- Who are you going to enlist as part of your support team for your first week postpartum? What would be most helpful for them to know? Have you spoken to them about the likelihood that the first week may be tough on you emotionally, and discussed what might help you during that time?

- What are you going to put in your self-care container? What kinds of things have made you feel relaxed, pampered, healthy and strong in the past?

- What activities have given you a sense of 'flow' in the past? Are these things going to be practical in your first week postpartum? If it is a very physical sport or involves trekking through the wilderness, it might not be appropriate during this week. Think about what types of things may give you a similar sense of 'flow' and be possible for this week.

- What thoughts have you had about yourself as a new mum? After reading this chapter, do you still think these thoughts are true? Have you been too hard on yourself?

5

On Feeding Baby: Fed really is best

Oh, mama . . . here we go! This is probably the most controversial topic of motherhood, because we mums . . . well, let's say we tend to have *passionate* opinions on the subject.

To breastfeed . . . or not to breastfeed.

If you have spent time online in the comment section of any infant-feeding blog—and I strongly advise that you *don't*—you know what I'm talking about. It can get *ugly*. It can get personal. The 'milk wars' are unfortunately a major contributor towards new parent guilt, lack of confidence, postpartum mental health issues, and division between mums.

Of all the postpartum challenges that new mums shared with me, feeding issues were the *most* common. Some mums were not able to breastfeed or had chosen not to breastfeed for many different reasons and were struggling with guilt, judgement and even bullying around that. Feeding issues broadly were causing so many of the mums I spoke to significant distress—some said their entire experience of new motherhood was affected by the struggle. Women were feeling like 'bad mums' because of how they were feeding their babies. Like failures. Their comments about the matter align with recent research findings.

A 2016 study indicated that the vast majority of mothers who didn't breastfeed felt guilty about that, and over 75 per cent of them felt like they needed to justify to others why they weren't breastfeeding.[7] This makes me so sad. It absolutely doesn't need to be this way. Women need support, not judgement. I so relate to these mums. I, too, felt this way as a new mum who struggled to breastfeed and switched to formula feeding within a couple of weeks.

To be completely honest, the continuous feeding debates I witness drive me up the wall. To me, 'breast versus formula' is a fruitless debate perpetuated by the media, and it distracts us from other, much more important issues. Debating the benefits of breastfeeding does little to help our kids, or ourselves. Rather than arguing about whether breastfeeding helps with things like bonding, intelligence, immunity, attachment and weight management, wouldn't we be better off using our time and energy to work together on ways to make systemic changes that we *know* will help with these things? Like adequate paid parental leave for everyone, affordable and good-quality childcare, comfortable living wages, an overall affordable cost of living, access to good-quality and affordable healthcare, and a great education system accessible to all.

Feeding issues, like physical breastfeeding challenges—pain, tongue ties, latching issues, infection—the inability to breastfeed for a multitude of reasons, or the choice not to breastfeed, caused mums significant distress and *guilt* postpartum. I was surprised and sobered to talk to so many mums who were harbouring guilt, regret or sadness over their feeding journey, even years later. I couldn't in good conscience omit these experiences from this discussion, but I do want to make a clear point here: I don't wish to be controversial. It's not in my nature. I *hate* the 'us versus them' divide that happens so often throughout early motherhood, especially with this topic. The last thing I want to do is exacerbate that. However, I do want to normalise the struggle, and to provide a balanced, non-judgemental and realistic point of view. Please bear with me, and let's stay friends.

To summarise my stance, I support breastfeeding. It is a beautiful, natural process that has been consistently shown through research to provide both babies and mothers with amazing health benefits. Breastfeeding is what our bodies are ideally designed to do. *However*, breastfeeding is not the only available option, and not even the only good option. It may not work best for every mum and family, physically, practically or mentally.

I also support formula feeding. It's a wonderful, perfectly safe—when there is access to clean drinking water—alternative to breast milk for women who can't breastfeed, or who choose not to, for a variety of reasons. There are many perfectly valid reasons why a woman may not be able to or may choose not to breastfeed.

My own feeding story is this. I hadn't given much specific thought to breastfeeding prior to having my son. I assumed that I would breastfeed him, but I don't remember thinking about it much. I hadn't heard much talk about it either, which seems crazy, considering the ridiculous amount I have heard about it since I have become a mum! There was a breastfeeding class offered by my hospital, but I never made it there, because I had been booked in for the class two weeks before my due date and, as you know, my son arrived five weeks early.

When my son was born, the midwife placed him on my chest to have skin-to-skin contact and to breastfeed, but I don't really remember this that clearly. I was preoccupied with my whole undercarriage being stitched up, which, as you can imagine, was fairly distracting.

Later I was given a chart. It had spaces to list all the times I breastfed my son, how long he drank for, and from which breast. I didn't realise I would have homework, but I was kind of starting to like the idea. I like lists, so no worries. Sometimes I even add things I have already done to lists, just so I can have the satisfaction of ticking them off. This one gave me something concrete to deal with, to cling to in a time of uncertainty.

A problematic pattern, though, was emerging, which I could see because I was so very conscientious with my list. This list . . . well, it was showing me a picture I did not like: my son wasn't drinking much—not as much as he should have been, anyway. There were no specific issues caused by him being born early, but he was only little, and not that strong. He kept falling asleep the instant I tried to feed him.

The midwives showed me again and again how to 'latch' him onto my breast and how to wake him up to feed—cold washcloth, tickle his feet, take his clothes off. They each taught me a different position to try. It was like learning yoga—footballer's pose, involving me tucking him under my arm like a football; the lying-down pose, which is what it sounds like; and . . . I can't remember the rest of the positions, but they all had cute names, and I couldn't work out any of them. I have an autoimmune disease that causes chronic joint inflammation and pain, and it was agony trying to remain in these positions, let alone manoeuvre my baby to keep him latched on and awake at the same time. Also, I have large breasts. I didn't want to include that fact here, because *how embarrassing,* but at the same time it was an issue for me, and I want to give the whole picture, warts and all. (That's a bad example; makes it sound like I have warts on my breasts. I don't. Stretch marks, yes. Anyway . . .) One of the midwives at the hospital told me that if she couldn't get me to breastfeed she was a 'failure' because my nipples were 'perfect'—*blush*—but I didn't feel like that was the case, because my son could barely fit his tiny mouth around them. I was in constant pain from trying to hold my son in these positions, keeping him awake and latched on, and at the same time trying not to suffocate his tiny face with my breasts. Big boobs can be severely over-rated while breastfeeding.

Over the next two weeks my son lost weight, lost some more weight, and then put on some weight, but not enough. He was diagnosed as 'failure to thrive' by the midwife who visited us at home and weighed and measured him. Whether it was because of my inability to do the poses properly, his tiny premature mouth versus my enormous boobs, his sleepiness, or an actual lack of milk—or a combination of all these things—he was not drinking enough. Because he was not drinking much, my breasts weren't getting the message to produce enough milk for him—breasts produce milk in proportion to what a child drinks, a quite amazing supply-and-demand type of cycle. Mine were getting the message that my son did not need them—perhaps they felt unwanted and were playing it cool?

I tried expressing milk, using an electric breast pump, but each day after hours upon hours of pumping I only produced around 30 millilitres, which was not nearly enough. Many women don't have any problem producing milk with a pump but a lot of the women I spoke to did, like me. They are not as efficient at removing milk from a breast as a baby is, and they frequently do not trigger the let-down reflex like a baby does. The let-down reflex is when your baby triggers nerves in the nipple, which causes hormones—prolactin, which acts on the milk making tissues, and oxytocin, which 'pushes out' or lets down the milk—to be released into your bloodstream. I don't think I ever had a true let-down. My lack of one may have been to do with how stressed I was becoming about not being able to provide breast milk for my son.

As you can see, I wasn't having an easy time with breastfeeding. I saw a lactation consultant, who told me that I absolutely had to learn to breastfeed and that there simply was no alternative.

'What about formula?' I ventured, hesitantly.

I was given a stern look. Anything good I had ever heard about formula, she lectured, was because of the formula companies' 'excellent marketing'. She called formula 'poison', and asked if I would really do that to my 'sweet boy'. (Spoiler alert: I did.) She told me that she had a three-year-old and one-year-old twins, and she continues to breastfeed all three of them, sometimes all at once. (She really did say that. Even in my sleep-deprived, emotional state I remember thinking, 'Wait . . . All at once? Does she have three boobs?')

Hearing her opinions as a first-time mum was hard. It was hard for my husband, too. We believed her. We didn't know any better. Neither of us had heard anything specific about formula, despite their alleged excellent marketing campaigns. It just wasn't on our radar pre-parenthood. So, I kept breastfeeding, in horrible pain—my usual joint pain, but also pain from cracked, bleeding nipples because by then I was spending most of every day either breastfeeding or hooked up to a breast pump. I was miserable. I thought I'd failed at being a mum before I'd even got going. How could I ever be a mum to my son if I couldn't even feed him? I had become a bad mum before my first month was up.

One day, as I was sobbing on the couch, my husband said, 'Enough!' He went to the chemist and bought a tin of formula. I felt so relieved and *heard* by my husband when he did that. Our son drank his first bottle hungrily, became much happier and more lively, and finally put on some weight, and from then on I was a bottle-feeding mum.

Looking back, I could have 'mix-fed'—supplemented with formula while also breastfeeding the little amounts I could. This would have allowed me to continue breastfeeding and provide my son and myself with the benefits associated with it, while also assuring that my son wasn't, you know, starving. I believe that with the stress and pressure taken off me by adding formula to the mix, my milk production may have increased, and I perhaps would have breastfed for much longer than I did. But I didn't even consider that possibility. Blame hormones and sleep deprivation, or just a lack of education, but it wasn't presented to me as an option. My humble opinion is that it should be. Formula, I found, was very frowned upon by the midwives in my area; the doctors, not so much—they were very supportive of my transition to bottle-feeding. But no one mentioned that I could do both.

If I could go back with what I know now, I probably would have chosen to mix-feed. Not only are there proven health benefits of breastfeeding for babies and mums—though, as will be discussed, the range of benefits is somewhat smaller than once thought—it also generally costs less money—note, I say less, not none, as the breastfeeding paraphernalia can really add up, and your own time is worth something too. Also, breastfeeding doesn't require getting up in the middle of the night to wash, sterilise and heat up bottles, which I loved doing—not.

I got a fair bit of grief for bottle-feeding. My family and friends were supportive. None of them said a single negative word about it. In fact, most didn't say a single word about it full stop, because it was a non-issue for them. My main problem was strangers, whose opinions shouldn't have mattered to me, but did. Several times I was questioned directly by random strangers on my 'choice' to bottle-feed. Once, when I reassured a lady at the chemist that my formula-fed son was in fact 'fine', she countered with, 'If it were me, I'd be aiming for a bit higher than just *fine* for *my* kids'. This kind of thing really affected me at the time. I began to feel self-conscious taking out bottles in public, wondering when someone was going to approach me and how I was going to handle it this time. I would make up conversations with people in my mind, preparing my responses, even on days when no one took a second look at me. (I had some great comebacks in imagination-land.)

I've had many breastfeeding mums tell me that they feel self-conscious breastfeeding in public. Some of them had been approached and told that feeding in public is 'inappropriate' or asked to go elsewhere. One mum I spoke to was asked to leave a coffee shop when a customer complained! I guess, once we become parents, whatever we do we can't win, huh?

I started to review the research on formula feeding and breastfeeding. I wanted to make sure I wasn't damaging my son somehow! I knew what the lactation consultant had told me, what I kept hearing from well-meaning strangers, and what I was seeing on internet forums, but what I saw in my son and other kids (and adults) who I knew had been formula-fed just wasn't lining up.

I found out that, as the lactation consultant had said, the World Health Organization (WHO) says that 'breast is best' for babies and breast milk is recommended for babies where possible. It's a natural, very healthy, amazing superfood. It has been linked with so many benefits for both mum and bub. It also changes composition, depending on what baby needs at their age, time of day or even illness, and it is just incredible the way the body can do that!

But I also learned that formula is a very good alternative, especially in Western countries with clean drinking water, and not at all poisonous. Formula-fed babies do incredibly well. Formula is different from breast milk, but not bad. We are so lucky in this country to have two perfectly wonderful and safe options for infant feeding. In fact, scientists have recently begun to re-evaluate the findings from previous observational studies supporting the 'breast is best' claim.

For decades, research had consistently shown that breastfeeding had significantly positive outcomes for children in many areas of life, like intelligence, weight, allergies, behaviour and immunity.[8] Recently though, researchers have found that there were a lot of 'confounding variables' in those studies. Confounding variables are things that skew the data. In the case of breastfeeding studies, these variables include social, economic and cultural factors. When the confounding variables were controlled for, some of the positive outcomes of breastfeeding went from significant to modest, and some of them didn't retain statistical significance at all.

A big problem with previous breastfeeding research is that the studies were mainly 'observational', which means that the researcher observes people and relies on things like self-reports, without doing any intervention or manipulation. The gold standard of research to determine cause-and-effect relationships is a randomised controlled trial (RCT), which is where participants are randomly allocated to either a group that receives the thing being studied (in this case breastfeeding) or a control group that does not receive the thing being studied. For obvious reasons, practically and ethically, researchers cannot randomly assign people to either breastfeed or not, so research has been limited mostly to observational studies. These types of studies are confounded because formula-fed infants can be different from breastfed babies in a lot of ways apart from the way they are fed. Perhaps they differ in socioeconomic status, race, early return to work for mum, childcare, where they live, exposure to toxins, or myriad other things. Basically, exclusive breastfeeding is linked with several social advantages and some of the previously thought benefits of breastfeeding are likely attributed to a range of other things associated with breastfeeding rather than the breast milk itself.

An example of a confounding variable is a woman whose husband has a well-paying job, allowing her to stay home from work longer than a woman who is forced back into the workplace after a short maternity leave due to financial considerations. Therefore, the woman who stays at home might breastfeed for longer because she is home for longer. Her kids may seem to be in better health, or to catch fewer colds than the child of the woman who is at work. But this might be because the second child is in day care every day with lots of other children, and they are exposed to more colds. That would mean that breast milk is not necessarily the reason why the first child rarely gets sick. So the confounding variable is the presence of day care.

Similarly, the child of the woman who needs to return to work early may struggle with obesity when he is a bit older. This is not likely to be because he was formula-fed but may have to do with the food choices that the family make, based on their finances and time. So food choices is another confounding variable. You get it.

In more recent years, researchers have been able to control for confounding variables in two ways: through sibling studies and a large RCT called the PROBIT Trial.

Sibling studies: This involves studying and comparing children *within the same family*, where one sibling had been breastfed while the other was formula-fed, rather than comparing children *across different families*. This helps to eliminate confounding variables such as socioeconomic status and home environment. Sibling studies broadly have made it clear that observational studies in the past have been flawed. A clear example of this is a 2014 study where the same data was analysed using comparisons *across families*, which found significant benefits of breastfeeding across several areas; however, when the *same data* was analysed comparing siblings *within families*, a lot of the benefits all but disappeared.[9] This phenomenon is consistent across sibling studies.

PROBIT Trial: The Promotion of Breastfeeding Intervention Trial (PROBIT Trial),[10] unlike previous research into breastfeeding, was able to utilise the RCT method because people were not assigned to the groups 'breastfed or not', but rather to the groups 'provided with a *breastfeeding intervention* or not'. Because the breastfeeding intervention they used had already been found to be very effective, they were confident the RCT would be able to provide a good indication of the benefits of breastfeeding—people in the breastfeeding intervention group were more likely to have breastfed. The PROBIT Trial was another way to get around the issue of confounding variables, because people were randomly assigned to groups and provided with an intervention.

With these approaches to research, some clear benefits of breastfeeding remain. Breastfeeding was found to lower the risk of gastrointestinal infection during infancy, and of course none of us want to see our babies sick. This is always the case, but is especially important for premature babies or those without access to medical care. It also seems as though breastfeeding is linked with a modest increase in IQ, particularly verbal ability, though the results of studies in this area are mixed. I do think it's important to note that if a mum is struggling with breastfeeding, it is unquestionably better for the child's IQ and development for him to have a healthy, functioning parent than for him to have breast milk. Breastfeeding has also been shown to provide health benefits for mum, including reducing her risk of developing breast and ovarian cancers.

Some other previously believed benefits of breastfeeding like asthma, weight management, diabetes and attachment aren't indicated when confounding variables are controlled for, which is interesting. Though the range of benefits of breastfeeding may not be as wide as once thought, it remains an amazing source of nutrition for our babies, and it is recommended by WHO that mums initiate breastfeeding where possible.

The thing is, most of us here in Australia *do* initiate breast-feeding. I think that as a community we've got the 'breast is best' message. We know it's awesome, natural and healthy. But for some women, breastfeeding doesn't work out. It may not be physically possible, mentally possible, or it's not what we choose to do with our body, for whatever reason. While reproductive choice and bodily autonomy seem to be recognised more than ever today, this hasn't seemed to extend to the area of breastfeeding.

Formula is a wonderful second infant-feeding option. It's a fine alternative and won't cause any problems for your baby. You would most likely not be able to pick a formula-fed kid out from a breastfed kid in a line-up. (Why our kids would be in a line-up, I don't know; but it won't be because they were formula-fed!)

My humble opinion is that rather than spending precious time and energy debating the benefits of breastfeeding, we should spend it putting our voices together to make change. Let's work on supporting research that helps improve formula, as scientists endeavour to make it the best alternative for our non-breastfed kids that they can. Let's work on supporting mothers who want to breastfeed, in a gentle, informative, but non-judgemental way. Let's work on finding ways to reduce cancer risk for mums who didn't or won't breastfeed. Let's work on making systemic changes so that the many advantages that are associated with breastfeed-ing like race, culture, work, and socioeconomic status aren't an issue—things like sufficient paid maternity leave, flexible work arrangements, affordable healthcare and childcare, and education for everyone. This is what will elicit change. Endless debates and 'us versus them' mentalities never will.

I want to make another important point: physically not being able to breastfeed is *not* the only reason people don't do it, and they should not have to justify whatever their reasons not to breastfeed are to anyone else, publically or privately. I feel very passionate about this. I made the decision a long time ago to stop justifying my decision to people who challenged me on this. I think it is important we stop justifying, and that we stop normalising people giving us the 'breast is best' spiel, especially without them knowing our stories. It's not okay.

While I can personally articulate my reasons quite comfortably, and none of them are *too* hard for me to talk about, what about the woman who can't? What about the woman who has been raped, or had a traumatic experience and who is triggered and re-traumatised by someone touching her breasts, even her baby? What about the painfully shy woman who feels extreme anxiety at the very thought of exposing her breasts in private, let alone in public? What about the woman who has chosen formula so that she can continue to take the medication she would be otherwise unable to take, potentially placing her and her baby at risk? What about the breast cancer survivor? What about the woman with breastfeeding aversion who feels agitation and intense negative emotions when she tries to breastfeed, and doesn't know why? It may not be so easy for these women to articulate their reasons, especially to strangers. I feel incredibly sad, but also angry, when I hear that these women feel ashamed of their feeding journey.

Let's simply accept that fed is best.

Breast milk is amazing. It's cheap, convenient, natural, and has fantastic nutrition, gut health and immune-boosting properties. Breastfeeding can also provide health benefits for mothers.

Formula is also fantastic. It is nutrient dense, helps our kids thrive and grow, saves lives for those who don't breastfeed, and it allows our partners to have a turn at feeding our babies too, giving us some extra sleep or a break!

Whichever way you choose, or have chosen, to feed your child, they will be fine. I used to feel shame. Now I know that I made the right decision to stop exclusively breastfeeding. When we switched to formula it was time to stop seeing us both as failures—him as a failure to thrive and me as a failure as a mum—and time to start getting on with our lives together— fed, healthy and happy.

The thing that is even better for our babies than breast milk is a happy, healthy mum. Your feeding method is only one part of an entire lifetime of decisions you will be making for your family, and in the long run it's a small part of a big picture.

Breastfeeding mums

For those who are breastfeeding, I obviously don't have much personal experience with this, and I'm not a doctor or lactation consultant. But from the many women I have spoken to, and according to the research I've done, if you find it challenging at first, I'm assured it does get easier with time. The first few weeks are, by all reports, the hardest, as you and baby both adjust to this very new concept. For you, being the sole source of nutrition for another human, and for baby, just being alive and outside the womb in general. It may not be easy at first.

You may encounter things like engorgement of the breasts—this often happens while your body is getting used to regulating how much milk it needs to produce for your baby's appetite. Your breasts may leak, you may have trouble latching your baby onto your breast, or you may just feel awkward and uncomfortable for a while. More severely, you may develop cracked nipples or even a bacterial infection called mastitis, which causes inflammation of the breast tissue and is very painful—quite a few breastfeeding mums experience this. Getting mastitis does not mean that you need to stop breastfeeding, but many women do at that point because it is extremely painful. If you choose to continue to breastfeed, you may like to talk to your doctor or lactation consultant about ways to help you through it.

After the early weeks of breastfeeding, many women reported that it became more natural and easier for them, and indeed became a pleasurable and bonding experience. I compiled a list of tips I learned from the mums I spoke to, such as what helped them to continue breastfeeding, despite any physical challenges, if that was their feeding choice. I've included them in the 'Let's Get Practical' section below.

Her story: Kate

Kate had decided she would breastfeed when her baby was born because it would be cheaper than buying formula. That was all there was to it. But, as she started to research it, she found a lot of information about bonding and the benefits of skin-to-skin contact between mother and baby. She became more and more excited about her decision to breastfeed.

When her son was born, he struggled to latch on. He became easily distracted and broke his latch on her breast every two or three minutes. She had to feed him in a quiet room, alone, lest he become distracted and pull off her breast, which caused her a considerable amount of pain and meant he wasn't getting enough to drink.

He nursed every one to two hours, including overnight, and Kate was exhausted by this routine. She was also lonely, because she had to be alone while feeding, and she was basically feeding all the time. It sounded petty, but she also felt frustrated that she couldn't even watch TV while she fed, because of the distraction aspect.

After a few months at home, Kate needed to return to work. She worked in an office job, and she was happy that she could express at work using her breast pump, so she could continue to provide her son with breast milk. However, the pump didn't work for her that well, and did not remove milk from her breast as efficiently as her son did. She needed to go from three pumping sessions per day to five, and it was starting to affect how she did her job. She nearly stopped pumping at that stage but decided to give it one more week, and then her milk flow improved. She says what kept her going was her commitment to breastfeeding, and the fact that she felt so strongly about it.

Now that she is nearly done with breastfeeding and pumping—her son is sixteen months old—she is both relieved and sad about it. Kate says that while breastfeeding was more challenging than she expected and did leave her exhausted and at times lonely and frustrated, she is glad that she stuck with it.

Her story: Amanda

Amanda gave birth two years ago and she couldn't breastfeed her son. She wanted to and did try. She checked with the lactation consultant at the hospital where her baby was born, and she was told that her milk would come in soon. When Amanda's son was four days old, and her milk still had not arrived, she began to panic.

Amanda says that her lactation consultant left her with reading material on the benefits of breastfeeding, and how the baby's intelligence and health would be affected if she did not breastfeed him. This worried Amanda, who was trying hard to breastfeed and had had no luck with it so far.

Amanda kept trying to breastfeed for a week until she was eventually assessed by a doctor who prescribed that Amanda take a herb called fenugreek, which is supposed to help boost milk production. It worked, a bit, but she was still only producing tiny amounts of milk, not enough to feed her son, who was proving to be quite a hungry baby. She breastfed and pumped milk constantly, trying to boost her supply, but to no avail.

She was eventually diagnosed as having low levels of prolactin, which is the hormone that stimulates milk production. Amanda wishes that she had found that out earlier. Then, she reflects, she would have spent the early weeks of her son's life cuddling and bonding with him, rather than hooked up to a pump and worrying about her milk supply. She added formula to his diet and continued to breastfeed him as well. He is a healthy and thriving toddler now, and she says that she never regrets the decision to feed him formula, as well as continue breastfeeding, only that she didn't start sooner.

Her story: Joanne

Joanne had always been shy. She always wore a T-shirt and board shorts at the pool and at the beach. Her husband lovingly teases her when they go out and she asks if her shirt is 'too revealing', because she has never dressed that way in her life. Joanne recalls being shy ever since she was a young child. Her mum had told her that a family friend sexually abused her when she was a young toddler. She doesn't have any memory of that, and she doesn't know if that is why she is shy. She just knows she has been shy for as long as she can remember.

She had a panic attack when she was pregnant, when the thought of breastfeeding entered her mind. Joanne felt short of breath, sweaty and dizzy. The thought and mental image of breastfeeding triggered an anxiety reaction in her, and it continued to happen each time the subject came up, either in her own mind, or through someone else mentioning it. She spoke with her GP, who prescribed her some medication to help with her anxiety. Joanne, her partner, and their GP came up with a course of action: she was going to feed her baby formula from the beginning.

When she got to the hospital, Joanne felt a lot of pressure to breastfeed. The midwife told her all about the benefits of breast-feeding and listed the 'dangers' associated with formula. The midwife placed her baby girl on her chest to feed, despite Joanne's protests, at one stage even grabbing her breast and latching the baby onto it so she could 'see how easy it is'. Joanne and her husband had explained their plans to the midwife, but Joanne, being a very shy and private person, didn't want to tell her about the abuse or her reasons for her feeding choice. She didn't feel safe or that she could trust this person with her story. She felt violated, and extremely anxious.

The midwife summoned a lactation consultant, who reiterated the 'breast is best' message to Joanne. She began to panic more when the pair told her that they weren't allowed to give her baby formula while at hospital, according to their policy. Joanne had brought her own formula and was able to feed the baby with it, but she left the hospital feeling confused, anxious and angry.

Joanne continued to formula feed her baby until she turned one. She doesn't have any regrets about the way she chose to feed her baby, and quite enjoyed the bonding time she had feeding her with the bottle. She vividly remembers the way she felt after leaving the hospital though, and feels it took away from the enjoyment of her first day of motherhood. She described it as feeling disempowered from the beginning.

Let's get practical

Here are some ideas that I hope may help you on your feeding journey, whatever your journey may be. Remember, above all, it is *your* journey, with your baby. You do what feels right. If your baby is being fed, you are doing great. Go, you!

Attend a class

There are breastfeeding classes held through most Australian hospitals. They can be very informative regarding the benefits of breastfeeding and the 'how to' aspects. You might like to check one out before having your baby, particularly if you are planning to breastfeed. As you know, being prepared and having realistic expectations about things can lead to more positive outcomes! In this case, knowledge about the ins and outs of breastfeeding may help with nerves and make mums more relaxed and confident while breastfeeding, which could contribute to having an easier time with the let-down reflex talked about earlier, which can be impeded by stress and tension.

Have a feeding plan

Like having a birth plan, you can plan for how you would like to feed your baby. You may have strong reasons for wanting to breastfeed, or strong reasons for wanting to formula feed or to do a mix of both. What is most important is that you feel comfortable with the decision you have made, and that it is right for you and your family. But, as with the birth plan, hold your plans loosely and be prepared to be flexible. Our bodies do not always do as they are supposed to, and neither do our babies! Our situations and even wants and needs, sometimes change. There is no shame in changing your mind, or in going down a new, unexpected path if you choose to or if necessity dictates it. Be aware though, that most hospitals in Australia will encourage you to try to breastfeed, at least at first.

If you have reasons for not breastfeeding and want to make these known to the hospital staff, make sure you have them written down. Sometimes it can be hard to articulate our needs, particularly when we are sleep deprived, nervous or overwhelmed. You don't have to disclose anything you are not comfortable with, and you are free to make your own choices with your body at any time, explanation or no explanation. Hospitals should respect that, but in speaking to lots of mums (including myself) it can be quite confronting to deal with what can come across as very strong advice in favour of breastfeeding, especially when you are in a vulnerable position; for example, lying flat on a hospital bed with a strange midwife's hands on your breasts. It may be a good idea to have on hand an advocate—a partner, family member or friend perhaps—who you have told about your plans and who can help you communicate your wishes to the staff if required.

Review the research

If you have struggled to breastfeed or have made the choice not to for whatever reason, it might help you to review current research on the matter. Formula has been found to be a great, safe alternative to breast milk and, after accounting for the confounding variables in previous research, there are clear benefits to breastfeeding, but there is little difference in long-term outcomes for children between the two. If you are unsure about your decision, it may help you to know that. Breast milk is great, and so is formula.

In doing your research, though, I would advise you to stay off internet forums on this topic. Those places can be *nasty*. They can get, shall we say, very personal. If you are reading articles online . . . stay away from the comments. I repeat: DO NOT READ THE COMMENTS. Seriously. Don't read them.

Consult an expert

If you are struggling to breastfeed, but want to continue, consult a doctor or an international board-certified lactation consultant, or IBCLC. They may help with your baby's latch, assess her for a tongue tie (which might be proving problematic for feeding), help with ways to boost your milk supply, or just assist you with whatever your personal challenge is. Your hospital should be able to provide you with some names of IBCLC. If you are physically unable to breastfeed, or it has been too long and your milk has 'dried up' but you wish your child to have breast milk, there are people who donate breast milk to 'milk banks', and if this feels right for you, then check it out.

Consider *all* your options

Sometimes there are feeding options that we forget about, or don't get told about in the first place. Don't forget, feeding is not an all-or-nothing decision. Many people successfully mix-feed—feed their babies both formula and breast milk. This may be something you would like to consider if, for example, you are not producing enough milk, but would like to try to breastfeed a bit. It is entirely possible to even just breastfeed for one feed a day. Many new mums are even unaware of the possibility of donated milk at 'milk banks'. Not everyone is comfortable with these options, but at least awareness equals getting to make an informed decision based on all of the options available.

Coping with physical breastfeeding challenges

- Be careful with your pumping routine at the beginning. Don't pump around the clock, thinking that your partner can feed some bottles and give you a break. This would be nice, but what won't be nice is your boobs thinking they need to supply enough milk to feed a small army, and then engorging to the point of near explosion.
- Wash your hands before feeding your baby, to reduce the risk of mastitis.
- Cold cabbage leaves are great for your breasts if they are tender. Keep some in the fridge, and then stuff them down your bra for a cooling, pain-relieving, day spa-like experience (well, kinda).
- Go to the doctor right away if you feel unwell. This should be a given, but you know us mums. We often get so distracted looking after our new mini-me that we forget to look after ourselves. Watch out for pain, fever, red marks on your breasts or any flu-like symptoms. The doctor may prescribe painkillers

and antibiotics—take them and take them all. If you aren't better by the end of the course, go back and get more.

- There is no shame in supplementing with or switching to formula. You don't need to put your own health (physical or mental) on the line to exclusively breastfeed. Formula is a fine addition and/or alternative.

- Enlist support. You are the main source of nutrition for your baby, but this doesn't mean that there aren't other things that your partner or support group could be doing to help. Consider what you need, and then let your partner or support network know.

Reflection

Over to you, mama! Let's think about you and your feeding journey. Grab your journal and consider some of these questions to help you work out what's best for you.

- Have you thought about how you would like to feed your baby? If not, have a think about it now. You may not have strong feelings either way and decide to see what feels right when you give birth.

- Do you feel prepared to feed your baby when he or she arrives? Would it be a good idea to attend a breastfeeding class, read a book, or buy some formula and bottles? Remember, preparation and realistic expectations are so important!

- For those of you whose babies are here already, how is your feeding experience going? Are you happy and confident in your feeding method? Are you comfortable? Does baby seem happy? If you answer no to any of those questions, would it be a good idea to tweak anything or seek help from a lactation consultant or doctor?

6

On Sleep:
That Holy Grail

Remember the days when you could go to bed whenever you wanted to, safe in the knowledge that you didn't have to get up until your morning alarm buzzed? Even then, the alarm had a snooze button. Babies do not come equipped with such a thing, or a volume button, or a range of Zen tunes. The quality of your sleep will now be intertwined with someone else's—someone who doesn't seem nearly as interested in sleep as you are!

No book about the adjustment to motherhood would be complete without a chapter on *sleep*! As the title above indicates, good sleep is the Holy Grail of parenting. But as you may have noticed, there are billions (probably) of books out there about how to help your baby to sleep, with a lot of, mostly contradictory, advice. Understandably, baby sleep is a big business! I would have paid a million bucks for a book that helped my baby to sleep if: a) there was any such thing, and b) I had a million bucks.

I am not going to attempt to reinvent the wheel by adding too much more to that narrative—sadly, I never found any magic solution for my baby's sleeping, except time and growth. Instead I want to mainly focus on you, new mum, and your rest. Of course your sleep is linked with your baby's sleep, but it shouldn't be *completely* dependent on it.

How baby sleep patterns affect you

Babies are biologically programmed to sleep more lightly and to wake more often than older children and adults. Their sleep cycles are shorter—approximately 30 to 50 minutes, as opposed to the 90-minute cycle adults have. Babies usually wake up at the end of each sleep cycle. Independent sleepers may put themselves back to sleep when they wake up, but it is common for a baby to need help resettling for a good long time after birth.

It is a false notion that babies will sleep when they are tired. They usually need help to fall asleep (that's our job) and the more tired they get, the harder it is for them to fall asleep. It is considered normal infant behaviour to wake up several times a night needing a feed, and probably a nappy change too, and then we need to resettle them to sleep, which is often the longest part of the process!

Usually babies tend to sleep for longer and longer periods as their first year of life unfolds, and eventually they hit the ultimate milestone (according to most parents): SLEEPING THROUGH THE NIGHT. (That required all caps, right?) The first sleep-through is amazing! When it happens. What if that's *not* happening, even as baby grows older?

In Australia, a 1994 study found that 28.6 per cent of parents had a problem with their four- to twelve-month-old child's sleep behaviour. Some 12.7 per cent of the children in that study woke up *at least three times a night*.[11] Studies found that a mum's temperament and mental health are adversely affected by her baby's poor sleep. Women tend to become more withdrawn and less emotionally 'stable' when their babies aren't sleeping well at night.[12]

My son didn't consistently sleep through the night until well past his first birthday. I used to be so jealous of my mothers' group pals whose babies, one by one, started sleeping through, until mine was the odd man out! He started sleeping through eventually, and now he's an *excellent* sleeper—which I thank my lucky stars for, because so am I! But every infant is different as to when they will sleep through the night and the journey is not always linear—infants go back and forth in their sleeping patterns according to stages of development, illness, teething and the nights you really want to binge on the new season of *This Is Us*.

As mentioned, there are lots of resources you can consult to help you with your baby's sleep—books, blogs, sleep schools or even sleep consultants who come to your home. These resources *may* be helpful for your family if there is a specific issue you need to address to help your infant sleep. Examples include establishing a bedtime routine, making your baby's bedroom conducive to sleep, learning good sleep hygiene—see checklist at the end of this chapter—or learning effective settling techniques—I've included later some basic baby-settling techniques to try, too.

It is important to remember that sometimes babies just don't sleep for long periods of time, for seemingly no reason at all! It may not be anything you are doing wrong, thus there may not be anything you can do about it. It may be something you just have to ride out. Believe me, that is something that I wish I didn't have to write, because it's a frustrating reality, but we are about realistic expectations, right? I hate to see parents tear themselves apart trying unsuccessfully to 'fix' what may not be a problem, but rather a developmental stage. There comes a point when we must accept that this is going to be our reality for a while.

We tend to try to fix our babies' sleep habits in new motherhood, but perhaps there is nothing to mend. It is completely developmentally appropriate for a baby to wake often. Some babies sleep really well from a very young age, which is also fine, but not all that common. Most do not. There is no such thing as a 'one size fits all' sleep strategy for babies. We simply need to take into account normal infant development when we are thinking about sleep routines and strategies for babies. So instead of trying to fix what isn't broken, we need to adapt our lifestyles and our own resting habits to respond to our babies' needs without completely losing ourselves to chronic sleep deprivation. We need to prepare, to be creative, and most importantly we need *help*!

Normal sleep deprivation

Most of us expect to be tired when our baby arrives. We know we are going to be up feeding them, changing them, and resettling them at all hours. But most of us have never before experienced the type of bone-tired, body aching, brain foggy, utter exhaustion that comes from chronic sleep deprivation. You have probably heard hilarious, relatable and even downright scary stories about 'baby brain'—putting keys in the freezer or leaving the house sans pants (points finger at self!). On a much more serious note, parents may be so sleep deprived that they forget their baby is in their car seat and lock them in the car, or they may roll over on top of them in bed. These are dark truths that seem impossible until you too have been in that place of chronic sleep deprivation.

It is important that we prioritise our rest, and seek help to ensure we are getting adequate sleep throughout the postpartum period. The reality of this in new motherhood can often be a shock that we haven't planned for. It's no surprise that sleep deprivation is used as a form of torture—it is really no joke. I want to work with you to manage your expectations around this, and to be able to maximise your rest and health, and minimise any distress and harm caused by sleep deprivation during this time.

Sleep deprivation is part and parcel of being a new mum. It is developmentally appropriate for your baby to sleep like, well, a baby. (How did that expression ever come to mean sleeping *well*?) Normal babies wake up frequently, with normal needs. Normal, normal, normal. The reality is, you are going to be sleep deprived as a new mum. Though frequent waking is natural and healthy for your baby—because their sleep is spread out over a 24-hour period, not just confined to night-time—it is *not* healthy for you, unless you have support to make up your sleep at other times. Chronic sleep deprivation can make a person quite unwell, physically, mentally and emotionally. It wreaks havoc on the brain and body.

We need to remember that while it is normal for our babies to wake often, until fairly recently it was also normal for babies to be born into villages, where there were plenty of people on hand to feed, settle and sit with the baby while the mother got some rest. Additionally, the mother wasn't also expected to go out to paid work or to run a household on her own. This village lifestyle isn't the norm in modern Western societies, and there are a lot of demands placed on new mothers with minimal help. Partners are often very helpful, but due to breastfeeding, busy lives and the partner's often-extensive work demands—perhaps being the sole income earner for a period—as well as societal expectations, mums seem to carry a lot of the baby-load alone in most cases, though not always, of course.

When my son was a newborn, I felt anxious each evening as the sun set. I felt the darkness swallowing me whole. I didn't know why for a long time, and then I realised the feeling was dread. The nights were so long and exhausting and I became anxious facing yet another night of sleep deprivation. Lots of nights I would sit up feeding my son for hours, tears rolling down my face, eyes aching and hanging out of my head, desperately telling myself not to fall asleep in case I accidentally dropped him or squashed him. Once he'd fed, he would take *forever* to resettle, because he had reflux issues, and needed to be held upright for a long time after feeding. I'd long for sleep when he was awake, feeling absolutely desperate for it. Then, when he was finally asleep, I would wake right up and not be able to settle down!

I guess I knew logically that my sleep would be impacted once my son was born, but I knew it on a very basic, academic level. It was sort of like technically knowing that giving birth is going to hurt, but until you experience it you realise that you didn't know the meaning of the word 'hurt' before that first push. I didn't know the meaning of the words 'sleep deprivation' until it gradually wore me down. Eventually I felt like I was living outside my own body—slower, foggier, and kind of unsteady all the time. Sleep deprivation hit me hard. Hit me quite literally when I slammed the pantry door on my face while I was trying to prepare a midnight bottle with my eyes closed—I guess I was just so tired I had forgotten to open them!

One day a friend came to visit. I hadn't seen her since my son was born, and I found I couldn't keep up mentally with the conversation. It felt like my brain was running in slow motion, and I couldn't understand what she was saying. At one point during her stay I forgot my son's name. That day really scared me.

Sleep is strongly associated with mental and physical well-being. When we aren't getting enough sleep, we are likely to experience changes in our mood, frustration tolerance, anxiety levels, concentration, overall physical health and a poorer quality of life in general. Sleep deprivation has been indicated in some of the largest disasters of the last 50 years, including the 1986 nuclear meltdown of Chernobyl. It kills hundreds of people each year on our roads. A research study in 1997 even indicated that it might be safer to be *drunk* than sleep-deprived once you hit a certain level of fatigue.[13] (Although I'm certainly not advocating that—don't drink and drive.) The point is, so much funding, research and raising of awareness has gone into eliminating driving while intoxicated, and yet sleep deprivation during early motherhood is not taken nearly so seriously. Instead, it is seen as a given, a rite of passage, and a competition of who has the funniest 'baby brain' moments.

Looking after a new baby, especially when we are just learning, is such a huge responsibility. In fact, I can't think of any other job where so much is expected of a newbie—and we are doing it while our brains are impaired! (Is it just me, or is that a scary thought?)

History has shown that sleep deprivation is serious, even deadly. During the early weeks and months postpartum, when sleep deprivation is often at its worst, we want to be in tip-top mental and physical shape. We are constantly learning new things, adjusting to a massive life change, and we have a huge new responsibility on our shoulders. Lack of sleep is not con-ducive to this, but we don't really have a choice in the matter, do we? Our babies are awake, and they need us! We are their comfort source, their food source, and their source of pretty much everything, in fact!

Postpartum insomnia

You have probably heard the sound advice to 'sleep when the baby sleeps'. A lot of mums give the obligatory sarcastic retort to that, along the lines of, 'Am I supposed to clean and cook when the baby cleans and cooks too?' Fair point. More problematic for me was that I suddenly found myself completely unable to fall asleep when the baby slept, especially during the day. Where once I could sleep anytime, anywhere, I now lay with my eyes wide open, willing myself to *just go to sleep*, and eventually nodding off just when my son's nap was winding up.

So many of the women I spoke to had severe trouble with their *own* sleep during the postpartum period. This can be a symptom of a mental health issue like postpartum anxiety or depression, or it could be a stand-alone problem. (Chapters 8 and 9 on depression and anxiety provide some effective strategies to help deal with insomnia, as it is a common symptom of both of those disorders, though it can present on its own as well.)

Postpartum insomnia is a real thing and many of the mums I chatted to experienced it. Research suggests that this could be because of hormonal changes after giving birth.[14] Women who experience hot flushes, depression and/or anxiety postpartum were particularly susceptible, and insomnia has been found to affect up to 15 per cent of new mums. When a person suffers from insomnia, her mental health, physical health and cognitive functioning are all impacted, so it is important to treat insomnia as a serious issue in new mums.

Some of the mums I spoke to admitted they felt like their whole world would be okay again if they could just get one full night's sleep. So we need to prioritise our sleep, and begin treatment for poor sleep and insomnia as soon as we notice it's an issue. Often we mums see sleep as a luxury, like a massage or a hot bath, but it's a necessity, like adequate nutrition and physical exercise.

Her story: Heather

Heather, a 31-year-old, had been working as a nurse for ten years. With no kids, she was often put on the night shift, and didn't really mind it. She adapted well during that time to changes in her sleep patterns and could sleep well at pretty much any time of the day. She was also used to frequent wake-ups and needing to function right away, due to being constantly on-call. Therefore, she was not overly concerned about any pending changes to her sleeping pattern when she found out she was having a baby, even as a single mum.

Once her daughter was born, Heather found that it was different than she expected. At first, she was unable to wind down, and lay there for hours trying to get to sleep. She said that she wasn't tired at the right times, and she was *really* tired at the wrong times. She tried to adapt to her baby's schedule, but her body, always so adaptable before, was not allowing that. She found herself growing more and more weary.

She remembers being stunned at her own swift and dramatic transformation. She went from being an excited, glowing, expectant mum to an exhausted, angry shell of her former self. She was so fatigued that she did not find herself bonding with her daughter. Instead, she felt resentment towards her baby, and felt angry with her for waking up yet again. She remembers one particularly bad night, when she yelled at her daughter, 'You're killing me!' She felt awful for weeks after that and thought she had probably damaged her daughter forever. She began to doubt that she was capable of being a good mum.

Heather thought a lot about the difference between her former shift-working self and her mothering self. Why could she cope with one and not the other? She thought the difference was the sheer chronicity of mothering. It was relentless. There was never any end to these shifts. There were no meal breaks or handover to the next person before knock-off. No light at the end of the tunnel. There was never any guarantee of rest or respite. She was always 'on'.

Slowly and gradually, over the first six months of her daughter's life, she began to sleep for longer periods at a time. The first time her daughter (and subsequently Heather) slept for a six-hour period, Heather felt like a new woman. She recalls how this happened once, but then not again for another two weeks. Two weeks later, these six-hour stretches of sleep became the norm rather than the miraculous exception, and she said she began to feel her body and brain 'healing from the inside out'. She felt like she was finally getting herself back. She was amazed at the way sleep had affected every aspect of her life.

Let's get practical

Have a sleep plan

Similar to a birth plan and a feeding plan, a sleep plan can help you to form realistic expectations about potential challenges you will face, and to plan ways to cope with these challenges. It's important to prioritise your rest as a new mum, as sleep deprivation is no joke—it can wreak havoc on a person's mood, concentration, memory, anxiety levels, anger levels and physical health, and contribute to long-term poorer health. There might not be much we can do about our infant's sleep patterns (remember, it is developmentally appropriate for them to wake up often), but there are things we can do to manage our own rest.

You might include various layers of village support you have in the plan; for example, what your partner, if you have one, family members or friends can do. Discuss the plan with everyone who has agreed to be involved. You might include, for instance, that Saturday morning is Nanna's morning, so she comes to pick up baby for a few hours from 7 a.m. to 10 a.m., while you repay some of your 'sleep debt' (more on that below). You might include that one night a week your best friend comes over and gives bub her 7 p.m. bottle and bath and pops her into bed so you can crash early. You might include split shifts with your partner (also more below).

Make sure you include in your plan the sleep hygiene practices (see later in chapter) you plan to implement, how you will set up your room and baby's room for the best sleep outcomes and efficiency with night wake-ups, and things you might need to buy—a night light for the lounge room, for example, so you don't need to turn the bright lights on, cooler sheets, or perhaps a white noise machine.

Split shifts

Many families, including mine, found it helpful to split shifts with their partners. My husband, a night owl, was responsible for our son's night-waking until 1 a.m. He would then sleep straight through until 7 a.m. to be at work at 8 a.m. I would go to sleep at 8 p.m., soon after my son did, safe in the knowledge that I didn't need to wake up until at least 1 a.m., usually closer to 2 a.m. or even 3 a.m., depending on when bub had woken up for hubby. This worked well for us once we eventually figured it out! We both got a long(ish) stretch of sleep and we were able to relax enough to fall asleep because we weren't 'on-call'. Of course, this is only possible if your baby takes a bottle, either of formula or expressed breast milk. If the baby doesn't take a bottle, then you may split tasks differently. For instance, a breastfeeding mother may be given additional breaks to rest during the day between feedings where possible, or the baby may be brought into her bed to feed and then changed and resettled by a partner, which will give her an extra few hours of sleep at night.

Pay off some sleep debt

It's possible to repair some of the damage of chronic sleep deprivation by catching up on some sleep during the week—paying some of your 'sleep debt'. This might look like sleeping when the baby sleeps during the day if you are able to, and it may be getting support to have a sleep in or an early night as regularly as possible. You can work with family members or friends who are willing to help with this, and brainstorm ideas that will work best for your situation. Be creative! One single mum I spoke to had her best friend, who was a nurse, pop over to her home on the way home from her regular Wednesday late shift at the hospital. The friend had a key and would let herself in and wake the baby at around

10.30 p.m., feed him a bottle of expressed breast milk that mum had left in the fridge, resettle bub back to sleep, and then continue on home to bed. She apparently loved being able to be a part of the baby's life in this way, and to be able to help her friend, and this allowed mum to catch up on some much-needed rest.

Settling baby

Learn the most effective way to put your baby to sleep. What works for one may not work for another—babies are all different! Some babies respond well to shushing, patting, singing, humming, rocking, white noise or feeding to sleep. Others need quiet, dark solitude. If something doesn't work well, don't force it. Try something else. There is no shortage of ideas on the internet to check out, especially through some of the sleep schools' websites. For a more personalised approach, you can even make an appointment to attend a baby sleep school to help with this or to have a sleep consultant come to your home. Don't worry about 'making a rod for your own back' or whatever other ridiculous things people say—the rod would be your baby not sleeping! Use whatever it is that works for you and your baby, and rest assured that you will not still be rocking or feeding your baby to sleep when they are eighteen years old, no matter what you do now. Do what works!

Keep it simple

Give yourself a break during the day. You don't need to be pushing yourself to your limits, driving around the countryside to run errands and keeping a perfect house at this time. You may not be able to fall asleep during the day—if you can, then DO!—but this doesn't mean you can't rest and relax as much as possible during your baby's daytime naps. Though not giving the same brain benefits as fully sleeping, relaxation and 'wakeful rest' will help unwind your mind and muscles and may even lead to a sleep if you are lucky. Try reading, meditating, bathing or listening to music. TV or looking at your phone is likely to keep you awake, so avoid those activities if sleep is your goal.

Sleep hygiene checklist

Despite what it sounds like, good sleep hygiene is not about brushing your teeth before going to bed or having clean sheets— though these things are also very nice. It basically means learning good habits and routines that are likely to help with the quality and quantity of a person's sleep. Here is a checklist of some such habits for your perusal, and they might just work for you.

- Your bed is a place to engage in two activities: sleeping and sex. Use it solely for these things, and your brain will begin to associate your bedroom with sleep. Try to avoid using your bedroom for other things. So, no watching TV, studying or playing on your phone in bed. Reading is okay—it tends to help with sleep onset—just not on your phone or tablet, as the blue light omitted by these tends to mess with your melatonin (sleep hormone) levels and sleep–wake cycle.
- Set up your sleep environment according to your preferences. Temperature, light and proximity to noise are all factors to

take into consideration in your bedroom. It is usually best to err on the darker and cooler side if possible.

- Watch your caffeine and alcohol intake. Both can wreak havoc on sleep. Alcohol may seem like it knocks you out, but it ultimately effects the quality of your sleep throughout the night.

- Try having a bath one to two hours before bedtime, maybe with baby. Doing so will raise your body temperature and, as it drops again, this brings on sleepiness.

- Try implementing a ritual or routine around bedtime. This will give your body and mind the cue that it is night-night time. A favourite calming song, some stretches, writing in your journal, or a glass of warm milk are examples of rituals that may help.

- Have a regular bedtime and wake-up time. If you go to bed at the same time each night—preferably, if possible, when baby does—your brain will begin to automatically wind down at that time, and you will find it easier to fall asleep. Also try to keep a regular wake-up time—as much as is possible with a baby in the home.

- Try to reduce overall sensory stimulation during night-time wake-ups. For example, if you need to wake up to feed baby, try to keep the lights and noise to a minimum and avoid looking at your phone, tempting as it can be. Instead, read a book with a non-backlit screen, perhaps with a small book light.

- Try some yoga or some relaxation exercises before bed—perhaps as part of your ritual. (There's more about relaxation exercises in the postpartum anxiety chapter, Chapter 9.)

- Turn off all technology for an hour or so before bed.
- Try to get 30 minutes or so of exercise during the day, as this will help you fall asleep, and improve the quality of your sleep. A brisk walk with the pram is a good way to get your daily cardio, get some fresh air, and get baby down for one of their naps at the same time.

Reflection

You may not feel like doing this, because you are so sleep deprived, but give it a go as it may be of great help. As you write your answers down it will help you to think things through and find a breakthrough idea, even if your brain is feeling fuzzy.

- How is your sleep going? Any challenges?
- How do you share night-waking responsibilities with your partner, if you have one? Could you be sharing the load more effectively? Who else can help?
- Can you implement any of the sleep hygiene tips? What will be the barriers for doing so, and how could you address them? Perhaps through partner support, or pre-planning?
- Do you ever feel worried about the impact sleep deprivation is having on your mental health, or even on the safety of yourself and your baby? Do you feel comfortable to let someone know about this, and is there anything you can do to feel safer?

7

On Your Postpartum Body: Unfamiliar territory

Most of us know that we are going to put on weight while pregnant. It makes sense, doesn't it? There's a whole baby in there! But when we give birth, we can feel pressure to 'bounce back' and reclaim our pre-baby bodies, especially if celebrity magazines' 'How I got my body back in four weeks after baby' articles are to be believed—they're not. (How weird is that term, by the way, 'got my body back'—I mean, where did it go?)

So many of the women I spoke to felt unhappy or uncomfortable with their postpartum bodies. They identified issues like being unhappy with their weight and body shape, being shocked about various *ahem* body changes—think peeing when you sneeze—and their body confidence in general. Body confidence was identified in both the scientific literature and by real-life mums as a hugely prevalent challenge in the first year postpartum.

Having a baby is a huge accomplishment for our body, not a loss of it. But, it can sometimes feel like the latter.

Body changes

We don't usually bounce back as soon as we'd expect after having our babies. Firstly, it takes a long time for our uterus to shrink back to its pre-pregnancy size. It can take weeks for our bellies to flatten again, and this can cause us to still look and feel a bit pregnant—even without any 'extra padding' we may have picked up during pregnancy. A few ladies I spoke to told me that they'd been asked when their baby was due—one when her weeks-old baby was right beside her in the pram!

Secondly, often childbirth can change our bodies permanently. Our breasts can change shape, our hips and pelvis can widen, we might have gained some 'tiger stripes' (stretch marks) and even our hair and skin can change postpartum! One body change I noticed that was a bit random was my feet. Even now, over three years later, they are a size bigger than before getting pregnant. (Internal sigh about all my long-lost pre-pregnancy shoes!) All these external body changes can cause us to feel insecure about our bodies. It may seem foreign to us for a while, as we adjust to the new normal.

Don't worry. You may always bear the signs of childbirth—and those are *nothing* to be ashamed of—but one day soon your body will feel like your own again. It won't always seem foreign, unpredictable and out of your control. It gets better. I promise. Pregnancy and postpartum are a grind on the body and some days you may not even feel like you belong to yourself. In the first weeks postpartum, leaky and engorged breasts, a stitched-together vagina or caesarean wound, haemorrhoids and bleeding, on top of sleep deprivation can cause you to wonder if you'll ever feel physically 'normal' again. That stuff is not forever. You will 'get your body back' in that sense.

Bodies change internally as well as externally during pregnancy. The pelvic floor—the layer of muscles and ligaments that support the uterus, bladder and bowel—has been stretched for a long period of time. It becomes weaker, and having a weak pelvic floor means that it is less adept at allowing us to control when we open our bladder or our bowel—so we may find that we leak a little when we cough, sneeze or exercise. (It's so glamorous being a mum, huh?) This is usually temporary, but it does take some work on our behalf to strengthen our pelvic floor again.

Emotional eating

In addition to changes in the structure of our bodies, both internally and externally, and putting on weight during pregnancy to grow our babies, many women struggle with weight gain and poor health *after* pregnancy as well, further decreasing their body confidence. One common theme that came from the mums I spoke with, and occurred throughout my own experience, was having trouble managing what we ate during the first year postpartum. I first wrote about emotional eating in the postpartum period in an article for www.mother.ly and I was blown away by the amount of new mums from all over the world who identified with this issue.[15] (Most of the information from that article is included here, and you can check out the original article on their website.)

Eating wasn't something that I gave a great deal of thought to when I was younger. It was just a way of not being hungry anymore, and of staying alive. Food was fuel. As I got older and started 'adulting', food became more of a friend, an activity, a source of comfort or a stress-relief method. Food became associated with emotions, rather than seen as fuel.

Every other species on the planet seems to view food as fuel—a way to not be hungry anymore, to have enough energy to live and enough body fat to stay warm through winter. Humans are different. We tend to associate food with socialising, celebrations, comfort, taste, rewards and emotions in general. Which is probably why humans are the only species who have a pervasive epidemic of obesity, and lifestyle-induced ill health.

When I was a new mum, I ate a lot of junk food—think quick, processed, sugary, salty foods. I think food was a quick, easy 'fix' for whatever was going on in life at the time—a quick way to feel complete, to be entertained, to feel pampered, and to feel full, not just physically but also emotionally. New parenthood was hard for me, and food helped—in the moment I was eating, anyway. It could be argued that binging on food is the quickest, somewhat socially acceptable method of avoiding negative emotions. Some people emotionally eat when they experience positive emotions, perhaps to celebrate or be social, but that was not me. I was all about eating to avoid negative emotions.

Since I'm a psychologist I really *should* know better. (We're not supposed to use the word 'should', as it's an unhelpful thinking habit as we will discuss later, but there it is, in my brain anyway.)

I know about how addictions are formed. Gordon Bruin talks about it particularly eloquently in his book *The Language of Recovery*.[16] He says, we experience something pleasurable—food, alcohol, drugs—and our brain stores it away for safekeeping. When we experience an unpleasant emotion—boredom, loneliness, anger, stress, tiredness—the part of our brain responsible for our emotions, the 'limbic system', interprets it as pain and potentially threatening to our survival. Our brain tries to distract us from our unpleasant emotion by accessing the pleasurable memory and forcing us to crave it. When we use that pleasurable memory to distract us from our unpleasant emotion, a new neurological pathway is formed. Each time we distract ourselves with that pleasurable memory, the pathway is strengthened. Eventually, the brain thinks that the pleasurable memory is necessary for its survival and voila! We are addicted. For me, in my first year postpartum, it was to food.

Since having my son, food has become somewhat of a crutch for me. This makes sense when I think about the acronym Bruin uses to describe people's emotional 'triggers', those unpleasant emotions that cause us to crave whatever we are addicted to: BLAST—bored, lonely, angry, stressed, tired. I was having these emotions in spades when my son was born, and still to this day, over three years later, although some of the initial adjustment (aka shock) has worn off. Now that I am aware of them, I can control the way I respond to the triggers more effectively than before.

Those are some of the most common emotions that mums I spoke to described! If we are feeling these things regularly, no wonder we tend towards emotional eating. Let's look at those trigger emotions.

Bored

As a new mum, I became *bored out of my brain*. I was so busy, yet so bored. Everything was done in a never-ending, repetitive cycle of feed baby, change baby, play with baby, settle baby to sleep then start all over again. There are a *lot* of those cycles in a day! Many of the mums I spoke to felt bored during their postpartum period—although many spoke about this in hushed tones, and said they felt guilty for even thinking it.

Newborn babies are so cute, but they can be very boring. It's a one-sided relationship for a while there. There are several long weeks of nappy changes, feeds, settling to sleep, and bathing before there's even a hint of a smile—which is probably just gas anyway—let alone a conversation about world events. The days of repetitive cycles feel endless, and the nights . . . don't even get me started on the nights.

Lonely

I am quite introverted, so you would think loneliness wouldn't be such a big deal for me. Not the case. Loneliness is not the same as solitude. I see solitude as intentional. I need solitude. I crave it. It is me creating a buffer zone between me and the world. It is a way to recharge, to focus inward and ground myself. But loneliness isn't that. Loneliness is separateness. Everyone else is the same as they were; I am different. Everyone else is asleep; I am awake.

Everyone else is at work; I am at home. When my husband had to go back to work after two weeks home with us, my feelings of being lonely got particularly bad.

Anger

I am often prone to fits of anger. I think it is the way my anxiety manifests. Anger, and even rage, is *extremely common* in the first year postpartum. (Yes, mama, you are normal for feeling this!) The rages were particularly bad for me when my son was a newborn, probably because of the sleep deprivation, hormones, unrealistic expectations and phenomenal mental load cocktail. (Rage will be discussed further in Chapter 11.)

Stress

I don't think I really have to explain this one, as most of you are probably in the thick of new mumming right now! Your brain is constantly 'on'. Even when you are not with your baby, you are 'on' as a mum. You will never have nothing to stress about again.

Tired

This one has just been discussed in quite a bit of detail in the last chapter. I love my sleep. I was a zombie as a new mum on limited sleep, like so many new mums. Now that my baby's older, I sleep better. Thank goodness.

Those were just some of the unpleasant emotions that triggered me to overeat when my son was younger. The eating patterns that formed while my son was a newborn hung tightly for years and, if I'm not diligent, they can still tend to rear their ugly head. When I feel frustrated, tired and in need of a break, I'm likely to go to the pantry and look for something to crunch my frustration out on. When I get some 'me time' I do not feel like the relaxation can be complete without some chocolate to luxuriate with. This is all subconscious—I'm not aware I'm doing it at the time.

My goal, and what I would suggest all of us mums experiencing this issue should aspire to, is to 'weaken' the neurological pathways that have built up in our brain. To change our brains' default settings. Each time we make a better choice for ourselves, it stands to reason that the cravings will lessen, and we will become more in control of our eating.

Between the body changes (both inside and outside) that can't be avoided during pregnancy and childbirth, and the common tendency to treat our bodies poorly during the first year postpartum, it's no wonder our self and body confidence takes a battering.

Her story: Alisha

Alisha had been a yo-yo dieter since she hit early adulthood and got married. She had never had trouble with her weight before and she had never learned self-control or moderation with food. She had never had to. However, once she got married she found herself cooking bigger meals that she thought her husband would like and matching him plate for plate. At the same time, she was getting older and her metabolism was slowing down, and she found herself putting on weight rapidly. She became self-conscious and embarrassed about her body and began to diet. However, she was an all-or-nothing person. She was either on a strict diet, analysing everything that went in her mouth, or she was completely 'off the rails' as she calls it. No balance.

When she got pregnant, Alisha was only about 10 kilograms overweight. As her pregnancy progressed, Alisha began to put on weight, which she knew was normal. But she described herself as 'giving up'—because she knew she was putting on weight, she didn't even try to eat healthily. She said that she was so used to the all-or-nothing approach that she didn't know how to do health for the sake of health and not just for weight loss. She was unhappy with the way she was eating, but she didn't seem to be able to stop. She had never learned how to have a healthy relationship with food.

Her story: Tara

When Tara gave birth, she was reasonably healthy. She had always had a healthy appetite, and was never into junk food, choosing healthy options most of the time. She was always a busy person, with full-time work and a hectic social life. For her, food was mostly a source of nutrition and the occasional social treat. However, once she had her baby, she had a lot more downtime. She was used to running here, there and everywhere for her job and, suddenly, her job was confined to four walls. Life's pace had slowed down. She described the feeling as being 'trapped in a cage'. She became bored, frustrated and felt 'worthless'. She began eating her feelings. First, she said, as 'something to do', a source of entertainment. Then, as time progressed, eating became a habit. It also became one of the only sources of stimulation during her days. After a time, Tara felt empty if she did not have something to eat.

Let's get practical

Identify the emotion

If we are eating our feelings, the first step is to check what is on the menu. Then we can work out alternative ways to approach the emotion. Are you bored? Go for a walk or pull out a project you've been working on. Are you anxious? Try a walk, or some deep breathing. Are you lonely? Call a friend. You get the idea!

Eat mindfully

When we are eating, it is important to do so 'mindfully'. This means, being present and aware of what you are doing. Due to the pace of life for a new parent, it is so easy to eat in front of the TV, or while cooking up meals for your family, or in the car, but doing so causes us to eat way more than we would if we were to really be 'in the moment'. It also means our brain doesn't register that we have eaten, so we seek out even more food later. Try sitting quietly when you eat—TV off, phone put away. Think about the texture of your food, how it smells, how it tastes. Enjoy your food!

Look forward

Ask yourself if eating this way will make you feel good in half an hour? Half a day? Tomorrow? Next week? Sometimes considering the outcomes of our behaviours is enough to stop us from acting on our automatic impulses. Some signals to remind ourselves to consider the future may be necessary, since we will likely be running on emotion and not logic when we are triggered. Have some photos, signs or a support person to call if you need ideas to help remind you to look forward.

Exercise

Going for a walk when bored, lonely, stressed, angry or tired—perhaps with baby in pram—is another good way of weakening the connection between negative emotions and eating. You are not only weakening the connection between the trigger and the behaviour, you are also starting to create a new, healthy and adaptive connection—fresh air, sunlight, socialising and exercise. You will also be within less proximity to the ever-tempting snack drawer—always a bonus!

Positive motivation

Having a positive motivation for becoming your healthiest self is much more likely to spur you on to act and to stick with the changes you make than having a negative motivation. A negative motivation is something you *don't* want anymore. A positive motivation is something you will *gain* from improving your health and lifestyle. For example, 'I want to become fit enough to have fun while playing with my kids', or 'I want to buy a brand new, stylish wardrobe so I can feel like "me" again'.

Self-fulfilling prophecies

Have you heard of self-fulfilling prophecies? A self-fulfilling prophecy is a prediction that causes itself to be true, based on the nature of the prediction itself, and the resulting behaviour you engage in because of it. If you predict that you will always be unhealthy and unhappy, you are likely to be so. This is not an airy-fairy 'what I put out into the universe' psychic thing. It's because your *own behaviour* will cause the prediction to come true. You are unlikely to treat your body kindly if you hate it and think it will never change. If you start to love yourself, you will treat your body like it deserves, then you will become healthier! Consider this quote by Henry Ford: 'Whether you think you can or think you can't; you're right.' Love yourself and think you can!

Food is fuel, not a friend

Begin to think of food as fuel. For survival. You can enjoy it, but it doesn't need to fill any emotional gaps for you. It is not entertainment, or company or happiness. It is fuel. There is no need to follow any specific diet, expensive eating plan, cut carbs, cut calories, drink only green juice or go on a 'cleanse'. Eat intuitively. Eat when you are hungry. Stop eating when you aren't hungry anymore. Don't eat just because the food is there or because someone else didn't finish their dinner and you don't want to waste it. Eat the foods closest to their natural source where possible. They will fill you up and provide you with the nutrition that you need, so that your body is no longer hungry, sick and tired.

Get out of the diet cycle

Make today your last first day. A healthy lifestyle should not be a black-and-white, all-or-nothing approach. You don't need to be 'on a diet'. You don't even need to eliminate any foods! If you eat a Mars bar for breakfast one morning after a night of no sleep, it doesn't mean that you've stuffed up, or that you need to 'start again tomorrow'. It only means that you've had a Mars bar. Hope you enjoyed it. Now keep going with your overall healthy lifestyle that isn't always perfect and has room for the occasional chocolate bar.

Postpartum specific exercises

There are some exercises and activities that you can do to reduce the internal bodily changes that occur postpartum. I used to pee—not just a little bit—every time I sneezed, coughed, or jumped for *ages* after pregnancy. I kid you not, two weeks after beginning a program aimed to strengthen my pelvic floor, this stopped happening. I still do these exercises now, and the problem hasn't come back. Plenty of free resources are available on the internet—have a look at Pinterest!—for these types of exercises. Simply type in 'pelvic floor exercises' or 'Kegel exercises', or sign up for paid exercise programs to get you going. As you can imagine, it really helped my confidence to get rid of this particular problem!

Reflection

Go ahead and grab that journal. Focus on you, and how you are going to gain some control over your body and your health at this very busy and challenging time in your life.

- Are you confident with your body? Your weight? Your overall health?
- What are some self-fulfilling prophecies that may be barriers to your healthy lifestyle?
- Do you think you have a problem with emotional eating? If so, what are your triggers? What patterns have you identified while reading this chapter?
- What are some of the positive motivations you have for changing your lifestyle and improving your health, right now?
- What are your health goals? Weight loss, increased energy, stamina, strength? A happier, more stable mood?

8

On Postpartum Depression: The black cloud

Depression: the black cloud, the black dog, the fog, clinical depression, major depressive disorder. Whatever you know it by, you likely will either have experienced it yourself, or known someone who has. Depression is one of the least talked about, but frequently experienced illnesses worldwide.[17] The perinatal period is when a woman is *most likely* to develop a mental health condition.[18] Despite all that, there is still such a stigma attached to being diagnosed with depression. As a clinical psychologist, I am passionate about reducing this stigma and encouraging people to talk about and seek help for depression. It is a devastating but *treatable* disorder.

People tend to think they can 'tough it out' or 'suck it up' through an episode of depression, but why should we when there is help available? Would we 'suck it up' through a chest infection, or would we get to a doctor on the double? We are not embarrassed about having a chest infection. We don't see it as 'our fault'. We don't see it as a sign of weakness, or an inability to cope. Nor should we when it comes to depression.

Depression is something that affects approximately one in six women in Australia at some point in their lives. It's also the *leading* cause of disability worldwide.[19] It can be caused by several things—*none* of which are our fault. Some people have a genetic vulnerability or predisposition to becoming depressed. Depression can also come on as a reaction to a stressful life event or period, known as a stressor. Often it is caused by a combination of these two factors.

Like any other illness, depression affects us physically, as well as mentally. Our sleep, our appetites, our energy levels, and our concentration all suffer. Why, then, are we *so* hesitant to seek the help we need, or to admit we are depressed? Why don't we see it as a real illness? If we broke our arm after having a baby, we would be rushing to gather all the help and support we needed. Likewise, people would be flocking to help us. But with mental health . . . well, not so much.

Why the stigma? Especially for new mums? A recent study found that 74 per cent of mums did not want to admit that they aren't coping![20] Perhaps some women don't know what's happening to them. Having a baby is a huge life stressor and can be confusing. What is normal? Where is the line between hormonal/tired/stressed and depressed? We don't know what we don't know, and lots of people don't know the signs and symptoms of depression. Or they do, but being a new mum is so different from life before baby that *feeling* different goes unnoticed.

In the blur that is the first weeks and months of parenting, it can be hard to identify what is wrong, beyond 'something doesn't feel right'. Mums might attribute that to sleep deprivation, being busy, or a normal adjustment to parenting. If we don't know what's wrong, we can't seek help. But it's not that simple, of course.

There are other reasons we don't seek help, like unrealistic expectations—both of ourselves, and also from the society we live in. Societal expectations on modern new mums are brutal. I love this quote by Bunmi Laditan, blogger and author of 'The Honest Toddler'. I think it sums up modern parenting life brilliantly!

How to be a mum in 2017: Make sure your children's academic, emotional, psychological, mental, spiritual, physical, nutritional, and social needs are met while being careful not to overstimulate, understimulate, improperly medicate, helicopter or neglect them in a screen-free, processed-foods-free, GMO-free, negative-energy-free, plastic-free, body-positive, socially conscious egalitarian but also authoritative, nurturing but fostering of independence, gentle but not overly permissive, pesticide-free, two story, multilingual home preferably in a cul-de-sac with a backyard and 2.5 siblings spaced at least two years apart for proper development, also don't forget the coconut oil.

How to be a mum in literally every generation before ours: feed them sometimes. (This is why we're crazy.)[21]

Not only do we live under this vox populi, we are also expected to love every minute of it.

Society perpetuates the idea that motherhood should come naturally, that we will be in a state of constant bliss. During my first few weeks as a mum, people would constantly ask, 'Are you just loving it?' I'm sure I looked at them like they were crazy. I never replied with what was really in my mind: 'Nope, not really' or, on my more sleep-deprived days, 'Please shut up!' (Hey, at least I said please.) Everywhere we go, from social media to random encounters in the supermarket queue, we are bombarded with the message to 'enjoy every minute, because time goes so fast and they're only young once'. (I still haven't worked out if that is a threat or a promise.) Society forgets that some days, from the new-mum trenches, life doesn't always feel so wonderful.

It's okay not to enjoy every minute of parenting. There are a lot of expectations around early motherhood and it can be scary for mums to reach out for the support they need when they feel bad about how they are feeling. Our fears range from being judged by our peers to, at the far end of the spectrum, having our baby taken away from us because we are 'not coping'. So, when we do develop a depressive disorder during pregnancy or after having a baby—known as postpartum depression—we often tend to hide it, either because we don't understand what is happening to us, or because we are ashamed to admit it. The problem is, when we hide it we get our wish. No one knows we are struggling, including those who need to know about it to help us.

There is another reason people don't seek support for depression when they need it: a depressed person often puts herself last on her list of priorities. She doesn't feel worthy of help. This is a lie her mind tells her, a side effect of depression. If this is you, know that you are worthy of care—from others, and also self-care.

Postpartum depression or PPD (also called postnatal depression) affects between 10 and 20 per cent of new mothers—no small number. It's a significant public health problem, particularly apparent in developed countries like Australia. This figure is just those who have come forward and sought help. The number of people suffering is likely much larger.

One Australian study, for example, recognised that one of the limitations of previous research, particularly in Australia, was that the researchers were using 'convenience samples'. This means they were studying groups or 'samples' of mothers in mother–baby units, or at doctors' surgeries, who you would expect may be struggling, because they were found at health services seeking help. They wanted to know how women *out in the community* were dealing with the adjustment to having their first child. While the stats they found were similar to the 'convenience samples'—9.9 to 15.7 per cent of new mums experiencing clinical levels of depression after childbirth—they also found that 25.4 per cent of new mums were found to be 'at risk' of developing PPD. They may not have been exhibiting enough symptoms to be diagnosed with it, but they were on that path, and they were struggling. Remember, these women had not sought help. This is a massive concern. A quarter of Australian women at risk of developing depression after having their first child, and they hadn't sought any help!?[22]

PPD is like any other clinical depression. The difference is in its onset, not in its symptoms or the way it is experienced, except for the added layer of pressure that is present because the new mum has a new baby in her care. The onset of PPD is triggered by—you guessed it—pregnancy or having a baby. PPD is usually diagnosed within the first few months postpartum—officially, only during pregnancy and the first four weeks postpartum, but many specialist practitioners will extend the diagnosis up to a year postpartum, and sometimes even longer.

PPD is different to the baby blues that we talked about earlier. The baby blues is not an illness but a normal hormonal response, and usually it goes away on its own, not requiring treatment or medication. It usually disappears in the first week or two postpartum. PPD is different. It is a disorder, and it is important to seek help for it. At its worst, PPD claims lives.

It's important to note that everyone's experience of PPD is different, and the symptoms you experience may not look like someone else's experience of PPD. You may have just a few of the symptoms and not have the others at all. Symptoms of PPD may include the following:

- not behaving 'like yourself'
- a low, very sad mood, perhaps you are crying a lot more than usual
- feeling overwhelmed, like you can't or don't want to be a mum anymore
- not bonding with your baby
- feeling guilty
- feeling angry and irritable a lot, you may even describe it as rage

- feeling disconnected from the people around you
- feeling empty or numb, like you are running on autopilot
- finding it hard to concentrate, make decisions, or function cognitively in general
- increase or decrease in appetite, or significant weight gain or loss (could be either)
- loss of interest in things you used to enjoy
- trouble getting to sleep or staying asleep, or trouble staying awake (could be either)
- loss of energy and feeling fatigued
- loss of motivation to do things
- feeling as if your body is moving too slowly
- thoughts of escape or even of death or dying
- harming yourself on purpose.[23]

To meet the criteria for a depressive disorder, some of these symptoms will have been present for you for longer than a couple of weeks. We all have bad days and will have experienced some of these symptoms from time to time, but a diagnosis is only made if it is a persistent problem, not a bad day here and there. It may be a good idea to chat to a doctor or therapist about PPD. They will assess you and provide you with the help you need.

I wanted to add a point about the first symptom listed—not behaving 'like yourself'. This will obviously vary person to person. This may mean, for example, if you are someone who has always been very social and extroverted, and suddenly you don't want to leave the house, that may be a symptom of PPD. Or, if you were always quite happy in your own company, and an introverted type of person, but suddenly you can't stand being alone and can't wait to get out of the house every day then *that* may be a symptom. Two completely different experiences, but with one thing in common: the person is acting in a way that is not usual for her.

If you do find yourself feeling 'not yourself' or notice any of the other symptoms we've spoken about here, the best thing you can do is to let someone know. This might be a partner, a friend, or a professional, depending on what you are comfortable with.

Her story: Lynette

Lynette recalls a time when her son was about two months old. She hosted a morning tea for her community mothers' group at her house. Lynette said that she did this because the very thought of leaving her house was insurmountable at the time, and because her husband had encouraged her to socialise. She had not been sleeping well and had no energy to do anything and no motivation. She felt so lazy. Her husband thought this was because she had not been doing things she used to do, like socialising with friends, and that she had gotten into the habit of 'doing nothing', so she thought she would see if there was anything to that theory.

She said that she smiled and laughed her way through the morning, and that no one even picked up on anything being wrong. No one asked her if she was okay. She felt desperately alone. She felt like a brick wall had been erected between her and the rest of the world. No one would have had any idea—not even her husband—that the week before Lynette had taken a packet of paracetamol in a suicide attempt. This was when she realised that you cannot tell what a person is going through simply by looking at them.

When her group left, she sobbed on the couch for the rest of the day. Later that night she told her husband about how she had been feeling, apart from the suicide attempt. She still has not told him that to this day—she feels too guilty, and fears that he will be afraid to leave her alone with their son. She was proud, though, that she did tell him about her depressed feelings. She had assumed no one would hear her, believe her or care. She realised that wasn't true; her husband heard her. He is now a huge source of support for her. She said that their relationship flourished after that first conversation, and that her husband had confided that some of the ways she had been feeling were common to him as well. He got it.

Lynette eventually sought some professional support and was diagnosed with PPD. She is still seeing her psychologist, with whom she has formed a good bond, and who is looking out for her safety. She has learned some good strategies for managing her depression, her sleep has improved, she is eating well, and she is more aware of what, and how, she is thinking. She now has the energy, confidence and motivation to leave the house. She still feels sad and alone some days, but these days are now the exception rather than the rule, when it used to be the other way around, and she knows some ways to work through these feelings when they appear.

Let's get practical

As I said before, the most important thing to do if you are experiencing any signs of PPD is to reach out and tell someone. This might be a partner, a friend or a professional. There are confidential mental health phone helplines available too. (A list of some of these resources is provided later in this chapter.)

Please note, the advice and ideas here are not meant to replace the help of a mental health or medical professional. This is an overview and will hopefully help you identify whether you need help and to gain confidence to seek the help you need, as well as to get started with some ideas you can try at home. However, it is highly recommended that you seek in-person professional support for a more personalised treatment plan.

Treatment options

In Australia, the first point of contact for non-emergency mental health help is your general practitioner. (If there is an emergency, where you or someone else is at immediate risk, call 000.) Your GP will assess you and refer you to a mental health professional, such as a psychologist, as well as treat you pharmacologically where appropriate. They can usually provide you with a mental health care plan, which will allow you to gain access to Medicare rebates for up to ten psychology sessions in a calendar year (information valid as of March 2019), and your doctor and psychologist will communicate and work together to support you. This makes mental health support much more accessible to people than paying full-fees to a psychologist, which can sometimes be financially restrictive.

Medications

Medication may or may not be necessary in treating depression. Talking, forming new habits, and various cognitive and behavioural strategies have been found to create lasting change in our brains and bodies, even without medication. But for some depressed people, medication is necessary for them to gain the energy to even attempt these types of strategies and changes. This is where medication may be helpful—as a kind of mental jumper cable—and it doesn't have to be forever. Many women are hesitant to take medication while they are pregnant or breast-feeding and this is understandable. Doctors can advise you on what is, and what is not, safe for you and your baby. There are options, but speak to your treating medical professional about all of your concerns.

Talk therapy

Talk therapy is one of the most effective ways to treat depression and many other mental health issues. The most evidence-based and widely used framework for therapy in Australia is cognitive behaviour therapy (CBT). CBT is based on the relationship between how we think, how we feel, and how we behave—and how these things interact with each other. Specifically, it addresses how our thoughts affect how we feel, which affects how we behave, which in turn affects how we feel and what we think about. Clear as mud? Don't worry, as there's more on this later. Below there is visual representation of the cycle of depression:

(I note that the concepts of cognitive behaviour therapy and the ideas and strategies discussed here that align with that framework are well established and used by most psychologists. As we will discuss, Dr Aaron Beck pioneered Cognitive Therapy in the 1960s and this was popularised by Dr David Burns in the 1980s, when his book on the topic became a bestseller. Many mental health professionals since have contributed to the growth of CBT as a therapeutic framework and field of research. As such, the concepts and strategies in this book are built on and credited to the CBT pioneers in the field of mental health and to the many, many mental health professionals who have helped to make CBT what it is today.)

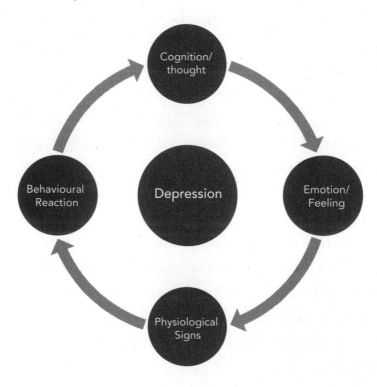

CBT should be used in collaboration between therapist and client, and should be based on the client's own treatment goals. It should also be used in a supportive, non-judgemental way. If you don't feel this is happening when you attend therapy, find a new therapist! For a personalised treatment plan it is a good idea to seek out some one-on-one support but there are some basic CBT-aligned strategies that you might like to get started with at home.

CBT addresses our thinking habits and our behavioural habits, aiming to improve the way we feel. It is helpful to begin the process of healing by implementing practical ways to change our behaviours and introduce new, healthier behavioural habits prior to addressing the major issue: our thinking habits. Behaviour changes tend to be relatively straightforward to implement, and they often result in reasonably fast changes in the way that we feel. This can place us in a better headspace to begin to work on our thinking habits, which can be very deeply entrenched. We will talk later about 'core beliefs' and the reason why our thinking habits can be so challenging to address.

Behavioural strategies
'Happy chemical' activities
To improve our mood, we must strategically engage in behaviours that are likely to increase 'happy chemicals' in our brains and bodies, improving our moods, motivation levels, sleep and concentration. There are four well-known happy chemicals and there are some ways to increase them:

1. Dopamine helps to improve our moods, concentration and motivation levels. *Meditation* has been found to increase dopamine,[24] as well as a *healthy diet, sleep* and *exercise.*
2. Endorphins improve our mood and energy levels, and give us a sense of euphoria. *Exercise, smiling, laughing* and *sunshine* have been found to increase endorphins.
3. Serotonin is a hormone that regulates our mood, appetites and sleep. *Exercise, a healthy diet* and *sunshine* have all been found to increase serotonin. Early morning or late afternoon sun has been found to be the most effective!
4. Oxytocin impacts on our moods, bonding with others, and feelings of love and connection. *Spending time with loved ones, physical connections, hugs, breastfeeding,* and *skin-to-skin contact* have been found to increase oxytocin.

The take-home message here is that diet—think fresh, nutritious foods like fruit, veggies, protein, complex carbs and good fats—and adequate hydration are important; fresh air, sunshine, and exercise are important; spending time with the ones we love is important; relaxation and sleep are important. Basically, self-care is important. Suffice to say, a walk in the sunshine with your loved ones, while sipping on a healthy smoothie = mood boost!

If we purposely participate in behaviours that help us feel happy, calm, connected and rested, we also increase our receptivity to the cognitive strategies we will discuss.

Getting started is not easy

Most of us know the types of things that are supposed to be good for us. The happy chemical activities, and in fact most of the common behavioural strategies for treating depression, are common sense, and nothing overly ground breaking. I always feel a bit bad addressing this sort of basic thing in therapy with my clients who are very much in need of help, as I don't want to make them feel worse, and you shouldn't. When a problem arises and we know what we *should* be doing, depression makes it almost impossible for us to actually *do*.

I can think of two possible reasons for this. One is that depression renders us hopeless and causes us to view things through a skewed, negative filter—we see ourselves, others and the world in this light and so why would we then have hope that these 'simple' strategies would somehow be helpful? The other reason is that some people are so deeply depressed that these ideas, which appear basic and straightforward to many, seem insurmountable. When we are depressed, we convince ourselves that nothing we try is going to work, especially not basic, common sense activities that we've all heard about a million times.

Exercise, a healthy diet, lots of water, plenty of sleep, social connections, relaxation and deep breathing. ('Oh, Miss Psychologist, these things are good for me, *really?* I had *no idea!*'—I can almost see clients rolling their eyes at me!) *But*, are we actually *doing* these things? Or are we discounting their effectiveness without trying them, because they sound too simple to be of any help with a depression that feels so dark, and we are feeling negative about everything at the moment? Or are we not trying them because they seem too difficult?

Above we discussed how depressed people sometimes need medications to even attempt any of the habitual changes necessary to treat depression. The changes might seem too *simple* or too *difficult*. Often we don't try the most straightforward and well-known strategies even when we know about them. We aren't *doing* them when we need to.

To be clear, I'm certainly not saying that these ideas are a cure-all for depression. I'm saying that, similar to medications, they are an emotional jumper cable, gearing us up to be able to tackle the deeper issues, the more entrenched thinking habits, the way that we see the world, others and ourselves. We need to be in a mentally sound headspace to tackle that stuff. It's big stuff!

There is a snowball effect with depression treatment as well. The most seemingly small change can kick-start a series of changes in an amazing way. Simply beginning a five-minute deep-breathing practice at night, and practising good sleep hygiene (see Chapter 6) may improve your sleep to the point where you have the energy for a walk in the morning, which helps your mood to the point where you call a friend, which helps your self-confidence, which motivates you to tackle a task you've been procrastinating on . . . The key is to get started. It doesn't matter where you start, as long as you start. Which, granted, is the hardest part. So how do we get started?

Activity scheduling

When we are depressed it's helpful to organise our days in advance and schedule some meaningful activities into them. This re-engages us in our world, increases our confidence, and lifts our spirits. Start slowly. Think of a maximum of four activities per day. Write down:

1. one pleasurable thing—having a bath, for instance
2. one thing that is good for your physical health—a 15-minute walk or a meal prepping session
3. one social thing—calling a friend, or sending a text
4. one thing that gives you a sense of accomplishment—paying a bill or cleaning out a drawer.

Scheduling your day might seem unnecessary, but it is one of the most effective behavioural strategies for managing depression. If this all seems like too much for you right now, consider just scheduling one or two activities instead. As I mentioned, the trick is to get started, and you will soon notice the snowball effect—one thing will lead to another.

Help someone else

Being overly inward focused when we are depressed is generally not a good thing. It's a common thing, but not a good thing. There is a time for self-reflection while depressed—such as when we are working on identifying our unhelpful thoughts and core beliefs, challenging them, and working through our own issues. We also need to focus on ourselves when it comes to our own needs and self-care. It's not helpful to be reflective and inward focused all the time. We need to frequently focus outwards, on others. This brings us out of ourselves and stops us dwelling on our negative thoughts and feelings all day, thus perpetuating them—like seeds, what we water the most, grows the most. Focusing on the negative increases our future focus on the negative. Focusing on others increases our confidence, sense of purpose and overall well-being.

Consider a way you can help someone else. This may be through volunteering, offering someone an ear to listen, donating to a charity, or whatever you like. You will feel better about yourself, and start the process of outward looking—this equals hope.

Practise being imperfect

Perfectionism is commonly experienced yet so dangerous for someone with depression, and also for someone in the postpartum period in general. Perfection is impossible. Trying to reach it will *always* leave you coming up short. Remember the Bunmi Laditan quote about coconut oil and other stuff earlier? You don't need me to tell you that that is an unsustainable way to live! As you practise imperfection—begin to value your flaws, and become vulnerable, not only with yourself but with others too, giving them permission to do the same—this will help you see that no one is perfect.

Cognitive (thinking) strategies

Our brains are weird. Cool, but weird. We now know, through modern science, that they change and reorganise themselves throughout our entire lives, as we learn and grow. It's a process called neuroplasticity, and it means that we can *physically* alter our brain's neural pathways by the way we think, feel and act.

One day after work last year, I drove home to the wrong house. We had recently moved house, and I had had a long day at work. Without thinking, I found myself in a completely different town from where I now lived. Whoops! Why did I do that?

When a road is frequently travelled, it is easy to drive on automatically. Have you ever arrived at work and realised that you can't actually recall the last few minutes of your commute? We are so used to our drive that we don't have to put much effort into navigating it. We do it on autopilot. If we are driving to a new place, on unfamiliar roads, with new sights to see, we concentrate more. We are more intentional and more in tune with the way we drive, and the direction we must head.

Our thoughts are like that. Based on our life experiences, and our interpretation of them, physical, neural pathways (roads) are formed in our brain. They are strengthened each time we 'drive down' these pathways. When we are depressed, by performing certain unhelpful habits in our thinking and in our behaviour we continue to think in a negative way about ourselves, others and the world. In a vicious cycle, the more we think these ways the easier it is to think these ways and the harder it is to break these cognitive habits.

To combat this we need to pave a new road—we need to train our brains to think in different, more balanced, rational, truthful and positive ways. This needs to be intentional, and will need to be practised intentionally for a solid period of time—until, of course, these new, healthier habits form new strong neural pathways, or roads. The goal is for you to travel down them by default. Remember, like seeds, what we water, grows. Our brains are amazing.

The first step in changing our thinking habits is becoming aware of what they are. Psychiatrist Dr Aaron Beck first came up with the concept of cognitive therapy and unhelpful thinking habits in the 1960s,[25] and it was then popularised in the 1980s by another psychiatrist, Dr David Burns, who discussed some of the most common unhelpful thinking habits in his bestselling book *Feeling Good: The new mood therapy*.[26] Most Australian therapists now base much of their work with clients on these cognitive habits, and many, many researchers and clinicians have since added to the list of common unhelpful thinking styles. So, you can find *heaps* of information on this out there in the world and the CBT-aligned information I discuss here is based on the work of many mental health professionals over the past half-century.

Common unhelpful thinking habits are:

- **Mind reading:** A very common unhelpful thinking habit, this involves making judgements and assumptions about what another person is thinking. As an example, a new mum might assume her child-free friends think she is boring now that she has a baby. She has no evidence to suggest this, and she is merely assuming, based on some of her own fears.

- **Magnification and minimisation:** This happens when we overemphasise the negative things that we do—or don't do—and selectively discount the positive things. For instance, when a mum completes only five out of ten things on her daily to-do list, she might tend to beat herself up over it, rather than feel proud that she did complete five things—no small feat with a new baby in tow!

- **Shoulding and musting:** Should and must are two words that really *should* be banned from the dictionary. They were probably two of the words most uttered in my early weeks of parenthood. They place unrealistic expectations and unnecessary pressure on us—or others if you are 'shoulding' about someone else, such as a partner or even a baby. For example, we may think we *should* have a clean house all the time and home-cooked meals every night. We might think our partner *should* be home from work earlier, and our baby *should* be sleeping through the night by now. This can be exhausting and even unrealistic, depending on other pressures we may be confronted with during the day. Life with a baby is unpredictable. We need to be gentle with ourselves during this very vulnerable time and give ourselves permission not to should all over ourselves.

- **Black-and-white thinking:** When you think in a black-and-white way, you are ignoring the shades of grey in between. If you are in the financial position of needing to return to work earlier than you would like to, for example, you may think that this is terrible, and that your relationship with your baby will be affected and that your baby will be unhappy at childcare. You may ignore the facts that you like your job, you are providing money for your family to be nourished and comfortable, and that your baby will have a lot of fun at day care and your close relationship will not be affected. In short, you will see only the bad stuff, but none of the good stuff, not integrating the two into a balanced whole picture.

- **Catastrophising:** This is when you jump to the worst-case scenario. If your baby is not a great sleeper right now, this kind of thinking will see you blow things out of proportion. You may begin to worry about the baby's long-term development or think that your baby will *never* sleep well, and that you will be tired *forever*—whereas the truth is that your baby is probably simply still learning to sleep and that the frequent waking is a normal part of a baby's development for now.

- **Emotional reasoning:** This occurs when we think that because we *feel* bad it means something *is* bad. For instance, if we feel depressed, hopeless or down, it means we aren't meant to be a mother, and that we are bad at it. Or if someone looks at us sideways, and it makes us self-conscious, we assume it means they are judging or shaming us, when they probably just really like our outfit.

- **Mental filter:** Having a mental filter is when you focus on and emphasise the negative parts of a situation, while effectively discounting the positive sides. For example, you take your new

142

baby shopping and it is all going well. When you are nearly done, the baby becomes tired, hungry and overstimulated and then, to make matters worse, requires a nappy change. Then, baby cries all the way home. Having a mental filter would mean that you dismiss the whole outing as a disaster, rather than realise that everything went well until almost the end, when the baby was overtired.

- **Personalisation:** When you blame yourself for anything and everything that goes 'wrong', you are personalising it. If, say, your baby cries a lot, you may attribute it to something you're doing wrong, or think that you are a bad mum. In reality, babies just cry a lot because it's their only way of communicating with us.

Do you recognise any of these unhelpful thinking habits in yourself? I know I sure do. I want you to note, though, that these unhelpful thoughts are common, and do not necessarily mean that you have depression. In fact, almost everyone thinks in unhelpful ways sometimes! This might have something to do with our core beliefs.

Core beliefs

Our automatic, unhelpful thinking habits are often the tip of the iceberg. I mean, they are what we can see, poking above the water. Below the surface, there are many layers of ice that we don't see, that we cannot touch. We likely aren't even aware that they exist. These are called our core beliefs.

Where do our beliefs come from in the first place? Well this is a huge topic, and it's not within the scope of this book to do it justice. I will just say that they might come from experiences we have had while we are young—often as early as childhood. (In Sarah's example below you can read an example of what a core belief might look like.)

Our automatic, day-to-day, unhelpful thinking habits are often built on our core beliefs. So, as we seek to change our thinking habits, we often need to dig quite deeply to find out why we tend to think in these ways and where those thoughts originate from. This is where it can be helpful to speak to an objective listener, such as a therapist, who may be able to see patterns and have ideas that we haven't identified ourselves. It's often difficult to work these things out on our own—we are too close to it all. This stuff is hard to work through and hard to change. Our core beliefs can form a central part of our identity and it can be scary to imagine changing that. The freedom you experience from working through this will be worth it, though.

Challenging unhelpful thinking habits
You be the judge
To challenge your unhelpful thinking habits you will need to put your thoughts on trial. You will act as the lawyer and the judge. Your job is to gather all of the evidence *for* the thoughts that you are habitually thinking and all of the evidence *against* them too. The catch is, there are no opinions, assumptions, guesses, interpretations, or conjecture allowed—cold, hard facts only. That

way you can determine if the thoughts you are having are true, or whether they are perhaps simply unhelpful thinking habits, that have been built up over the years, perhaps due to some of your past experiences and resulting core beliefs.

A good way to do this is to use this 'Thought' template. Draw it up in your journal and modify it any way that suits you and your thinking. Write at the top the thought you wish to examine and then fill in the spaces below. Remember, this is your journal, and just for you. (Sarah's story below, and her thought-challenging exercise, might give you more ideas about how to go about doing this exercise.)

The Thought	
Evidence FOR the Thought	Evidence AGAINST the Thought
The Verdict	

Behavioural experiments

Another way to test the validity of your unhelpful thinking habits is by testing them in real life—not just on paper. We can test the validity of our thoughts about ourselves, others and the world around us through behavioural experiments. These have the same purpose as the thought-challenging activity (above) does: they let us test the truthfulness of our often long-held negative beliefs and thinking habits.

We often have preconceived ideas or predictions about what will happen in certain situations. We can test these predictions like scientists in a laboratory. Our predictions about what we expect will happen form our 'hypothesis'. We test our hypothesis out in real life. We then examine the results and check whether what we expected to happen did actually happen or not. More often than not, a depressed person's outlook is skewed towards the negative and, when they test their negative predictions, they can 'prove themselves wrong'—in a good way!

Let's look at Jane, as an example. She feels depressed. She recently had a baby, and thinks that everything has changed. Jane predicts that she will never have any time to herself, and that the things she used to enjoy, like exercising and socialising, are things of the past. She thinks her life, as she knew it, is over. Jane sets out to test this hypothesis.

Hypothesis: I won't be able to exercise or enjoy time with my friends with the baby in tow. The baby will get bored, or need a feed, or scream and cry, and there is no point going out at all.

Experiment: Take the baby in the pram and my friend out for a power walk with a takeaway coffee. See what happens.

Outcome: Apart from one unfortunate nappy blowout, the walk was pleasant. I got some exercise and fresh air and was happy to catch up on some of my friend's news—we laughed a lot. When we got home, my friend helped me inside with the baby and we arranged to make power walking a weekly event. I realised that, though lots of things are different now that I have a baby, I can find ways to continue to look after my health and do the things I enjoy—it's a matter of finding the 'new normal'.

Sarah's strategies

When Sarah was nine years old, her father left her mother and moved back to the United States, where he was from. He didn't stay in contact. Sarah doesn't remember much about that time, but she thinks she has had trouble trusting people ever since.

When she was thirteen years old, she had a fight with her best friend over something small. Her friend was very popular and outgoing, and when they fought, most of their friendship group turned against Sarah. Sarah made a new group of friends, but wasn't especially close to any one person, and didn't maintain any of these friendships after she graduated from school.

After school finished, Sarah worked in three or four different offices over the next decade. She has always been easy to get along with and has never had a shortage of friends. But the friendships have always ended when she moved on from any given school or job. She has continuously felt 'on the outside' and never felt a sense of belonging in any group or in the world in general. Eventually she met her partner, and she says that this was the first time that she felt like she belonged to someone. After she met him, she started to become friends with his friends. She really enjoys spending time with them. Their friends don't have kids yet.

When Sarah gave birth to her daughter, she started to worry that her friends would think she was boring now that she was a mum. She worried they wouldn't have much in common anymore, and that they wouldn't want to spend as much time with her. She felt sad, angry, lonely, embarrassed and hurt. Nothing bad had happened but she *felt* like it had. She had the *unhelpful* and most likely *untrue* cognition that no one wanted to see her because they thought she was boring. This was probably due to her core belief that she is not worthy, built on her background story of rejection, mistrust and abandonment. She feared that she was facing yet another rejection. If his friends rejected her, might her partner realise his mistake and abandon her too?

Sarah experienced a physiological reaction: she had bad insomnia, she lost her appetite, was lethargic, fatigued, teary and unmotivated. She began to behave in a way that was unhelpful. She isolated herself, avoiding her friends' phone calls, said no to outings—even with her partner—and didn't respond to texts and social media posts. She thinks she was doing this out of self-preservation.

Unfortunately for Sarah, this turned out to be a self-fulfilling prophecy. Her friends had never thought she was boring at all. On the contrary; they were excited to spoil her baby, the first baby in their group. When Sarah ceased communication with them, they wrongly assumed that she had better things to do than socialise with them and, after a while, they stopped trying.

Sarah was once again left with minimal social connections and was feeling abandoned by the people close to her. The cycle of depression can be used to map out Sarah's thoughts, feelings, physiological reactions and behaviours. As we can see, they have a strong influence on each other.

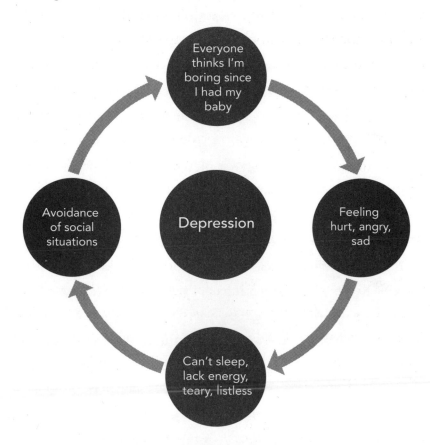

Sarah cycled around and around, and it was like drilling into a wall. The more times she cycled around, the deeper entrenched her thoughts, feelings and behaviours got. By engaging in the cycle, she was strengthening the negative neural pathways in her mind. She was clearing the path to continue thinking that way by default. She was watering the wrong seeds.

I think of it like this: You know that one instruction you get when you have one of those pain-in-the-bum flat packs to put together: 'Righty tighty, lefty loosey?' Going right around the cycle was tightening Sarah's thoughts, making them stronger, more entrenched and more permanent. Going left around the cycle would loosen them up, freeing her. Right was choosing to follow and strengthen the well-worn path towards negativity and unhelpful thoughts and left would be choosing to deliberately pave a new path towards positivity and balance. But Sarah needed to *change* something somewhere in the cycle, in order to reverse it.

I suggested Sarah start by looking at what she could do to improve her physiological responses—the physical, practical stuff. As we discussed before, it is helpful to begin with forming positive habits—working on sleep, exercise, diet and general self-care—to help increase her confidence, motivation and energy. Then she would begin to feel happier and more settled in herself. This worked well. Sarah then re-engaged in her world, attending some social events. She began gathering evidence that suggested that her friends thought she was fun to be around, and that she *was* fun! She then attended another function, gathered more evidence. She was now reversing the cycle and removing that drill from the wall. Lefty loosey. It looked like this:

Luckily, Sarah decided to address her issues in therapy, once she noticed the spiral she was in. Sarah began to feel more

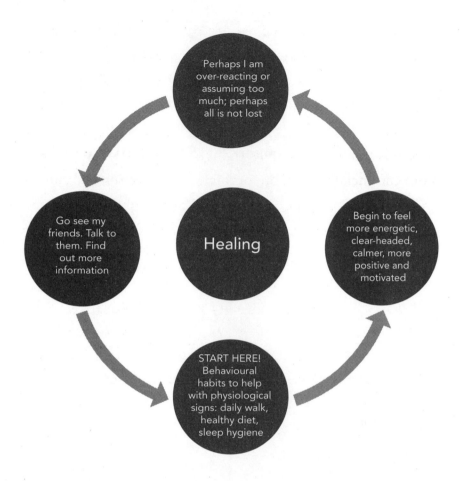

positive by practising the behavioural strategies, and re-engaging with her world, and then she felt better equipped to start getting to the bottom of some of her thinking habits. Below is her completed thought-challenging sheet. No opinions, conjecture, interpretations, assumptions or guesses were allowed in doing this, and they shouldn't be part of your thought-challenging exercises!

The Thoughts

My friends all think I am boring since I had my baby. I never fit in anywhere. I always lose the friends I find. If my partner's friends don't like me, he will realise his mistake and leave me.

Evidence FOR the Thought	Evidence AGAINST the Thought
No one else has a baby and I do	Jenny has called me twice in the past week
I've not been out of the house for a while	Kate tagged me on social media in a video about new mums and asked me if I needed anything
I'm feeling bad about myself	My friends threw a baby shower and bought a gift
	Jack (partner) laughed at my joke this morning and has never said I was boring or acted like I was
	I've always had friends and people to hang out with

The Verdict

I worry that people will think I am boring because I'm the first to have a baby, and that scares me. In truth, the evidence shows that people want to see me and talk to me, and think I am fun. I am worrying about this because I feel bad about myself and I'm scared, not because it's true.

As well as on paper, Sarah decided to conduct a behavioural experiment.

Hypothesis: My friends have all stopped contacting me, because I ignored them for so long. If I go to Jessica's engagement party with my partner, no one will talk to me and I'll be standing in the corner all night feeling awkward.

Experiment: Go to the engagement party, try talking to some of my friends, ask them how they are, apologise for not being in contact, tell them I miss them.

Outcome: When I saw my friends, I felt the urge to be honest with them. I told them that new-mum life was different than I expected, and that I felt self-conscious, being the first of us all with a baby. My friends understood, and apologised for not recognising that and pushing harder. At the end of the night I arranged to catch up with my friends again. I realised that my friends value our friendship as much as I do.

Helplines

All the ideas in this chapter you can either begin practising at home or use to gather information about what kinds of things therapy can help you with. I highly recommend seeking individually tailored support. Start with your GP, or one of the helplines listed below. They are excellent resources that will help you. All you need to do is show up and ask.

- **PANDA:** Perinatal Anxiety and Depression Australia[27] is an Australian organisation that aims to support new parents who are affected by anxiety and depression during pregnancy and their first year of parenthood. They have a website (www.panda. org.au) with great resources, and a helpline, on 1300 726 306, which runs weekdays from 9 a.m. to 7.30 p.m. AEST/AEDT. Consider giving them a call and check out their website.
- **Lifeline:** Lifeline is a 24-hour, 7-day-a-week crisis support and suicide helpline, for people experiencing a crisis or thinking about suicide. They are available all the time on 13 11 14.

Reflection

Grab your journal, as here are some questions to help you work through some of the issues raised in this chapter.

- Have a read through the symptoms of depression listed above. Do you relate to any of them?
- What do you think about Lynette's story, and how none of her friends was able to tell that anything was wrong?
- Is there someone that you feel comfortable talking to about the way you feel? If not, what are the barriers holding you back?
- What are some of the behavioural activities you could engage in this week to help increase your happy, mood boosting chemicals?
- Do you relate to some of the unhelpful thinking styles listed above? Complete the CBT activity in your journal.

- If the thoughts you identified above are not helpful, or you suspect they are not true, what is a behavioural experiment that you could try to help you gather more evidence about the thought to 'prove yourself wrong'? After you've done it, write down the outcome in your journal.

9

On Postpartum Anxiety: The cold mist

If depression is a black cloud, then anxiety, to me, is a cold mist. It sneaks up on you and it's pervasive, uncomfortable and chilling. It's like being Chicken Little, the only one who knows the sky is falling and no one believes you. It is living in a state of five-alarm emergency, when there is no actual danger. Anxiety can present at any stage in life, but it is frequently triggered by pregnancy, childbirth and becoming a mum for the first time.

I've always been an anxious person. When I was a child, I couldn't stand it if my socks didn't line up perfectly at my knees. As a teenager, I slept with a light on every night, and I wouldn't order a pizza by myself, because I was so scared of the phone. I worked my way up into a flurry before social events, and I overthought everything. This is part of the reason I chose to study psychology. I improved *a lot* as an adult, but still tend towards anxiety with certain things.

To be honest, I still don't swim in the ocean. A few years ago I thought how ridiculous it was that a psychologist living near the beach was scared of the ocean, and so I decided to get serious about conquering this irrational fear. My fears around the ocean were (are) many: sharks—actually, all living creatures—rips, currents, big waves, and showing everyone my bathing suit body. So, I summoned all of my courage, got into my bathers, marched down to the water, and went in.

So far, so good—for about five minutes, when a giant stingray jumped out of a big wave right in front of me. Hightailing it back to shore, I promptly bumped into one of my regular clients—yes, in my bathers. I haven't been in past my knees since. Luckily for me, my son is still small enough to swim at the depth I am comfortable at, but I'm well aware that this will be a fear I need to conquer as he grows older!

My anxiety was particularly bad in my early postpartum period. I worried about *everything* when my son was a baby. To a degree, parents tend to worry by nature and design. It's completely normal for a new mum to worry about her baby's well-being and safety. It's a survival instinct—some level of anxiety is adaptive. It is our job to protect our baby, our family, from threats. It starts in pregnancy.

Adaptive anxiety continues once our babies are born— buying baby monitors, following the safe-sleep guidelines to the letter, making sure our kids wear bike helmets. Anxiety can be a good thing: it keeps our babies safe. As new mums we tend to become hypervigilant, on the lookout for every possible threat. It's our job. It's normal to be anxious, and to worry about things, because we've just been given this hugely important new responsibility—a human life, for goodness sakes! When my son was a baby, I would see danger lurking around every corner. Each table had a potentially deadly sharp edge, and each staircase was a double black diamond run and a disaster waiting to happen.

Anxiety becomes problematic when the level of worry you experience stops being adaptive and helpful. Instead, it starts to affect your daily functioning. Perhaps it impacts on your relationship, your social life, your bonding with your baby, your work or your physical health. This is called an anxiety disorder, and there are many types of anxiety disorders.

The fight or flight response

Our bodies are designed to respond quickly and automatically to threats. When we sense that we are in danger, this triggers a physiological response: a torrent of well-orchestrated stress hormones that cause physiological changes in our body. Our muscles tense, our breathing quickens, our heart pounds and our pupils dilate. We call this the 'fight or flight response'. This coordinated series of hormonal and physiological changes has evolved as a survival mechanism, so that we have the means to stand and fight or run away from dangerous situations, like wild animals, attackers or natural disasters.

Generally, we are safe in our everyday lives in modern Australia. But unfortunately, our bodies haven't quite evolved to know the difference between a real, actual threat, like an advancing lion, and a 'perceived threat', like a funny look from someone in the supermarket, or a sharp coffee table corner. Just because the fight or flight response happens automatically, it doesn't make it the correct response at the time. The type of anxiety we usually experience revolves more around perceived threats than actual ones. So, our bodies are constantly responding, reacting as if they are under attack, when they probably aren't.

One problem with the fight or flight response is that it is only helpful in short bursts, for emergencies. It provides us with the physiological means and energy we need to fight or run away from a threat. We use up the energy while fighting or running, and then our body returns to its normal state. However, perceived threats are more of a chronic stress issue—we could be under this type of stress every single day, not just during occasional emergencies. We also don't 'use up' or 'burn off' the energy provided by the rush of hormones triggered by the fight or flight response during a perceived threat—because there is nothing to physically fight or run from. So, we are living in high levels of arousal, tension, and basically are in survival mode all the time, with no outlet.

Over time, this is harmful for us in lots of ways. We can have way too much energy to fall asleep, and once we do, we have trouble maintaining our sleep. Our 'less important' secondary functions, like digestion, are shut down because our bodies think they are in survival mode, and don't have room to focus on pesky little things like digesting our food, so we experience things like appetite loss, stomach aches, and toileting issues (those are fun). Our muscles are constantly tense, so we may get aches and pains and headaches. We basically become a big ball of anxiety, feeling unwell, fatigued, tense—*all the time!* It's completely exhausting.

People tell us things like 'don't worry about it' or 'it's not likely to happen' when we confess our worries to them. But the thing is, we can't help it! Our emotional brain (our limbic system) and our rational, logical brain (our prefrontal cortex) can't both be in charge of us at the same time. When our anxiety is triggered, our limbic system impedes our rational brain and, with it, our ability to think rationally. So, we need to calm our emotional brain down and switch our logical brain back on before we can attempt the well-meaning advice to 'just not worry about it'. (We'll discuss some ways to do this in the 'Let's Get Practical' section.)

As I said, some level of anxiety is normal, especially in periods of adjustment and change, like new motherhood. But an anxiety *disorder* is something above and beyond normal anxiety. It is more severe, longer lasting, and it impacts on our daily lives—social lives, work lives, parenting lives.

What the research says

While maternal mental health has started to gain a lot more attention and research over the past decade, much of the focus to date has been on depressive symptoms and anxiety has been somewhat overlooked. A review of the current research indicates that anywhere between 4.7 and 33 per cent of women experience postpartum anxiety—as in, increased amounts of anxiety in the first twelve months postpartum.[28] While this range is massive, and sounds like it doesn't tell us much, it does indicate that, regardless of the figures, women are suffering with anxiety disorders in their first twelve months as mums—so that's the important bit to pay attention to.

The large range probably has something to do with the fact that there is little consistency in the way researchers have been looking at this issue. Some of the literature reviewed, for example, was focused solely on specific groups of women, some on teenaged mums, some on mums who had assistance getting pregnant, like with IVF, or on mums with a history of previous loss—stillbirth or miscarriage. Also, some of the studies were done with convenience samples, as discussed previously—samples of women who had presented at mental health clinics or hospitals, seeking help for themselves or their babies. It would stand to reason that studies focusing on mums who were seeking help, or who had additional stressors in their lives, would indicate anxiety in larger numbers than studies that focused on the general community.

Mums across all walks of life are struggling with postpartum anxiety. The pattern across the research seems to be that anxiety levels peak at the very beginning of motherhood, which makes sense due to the massive adjustment we keep talking about, and then, in a lot of cases, levels slowly improve over the course of that first year.[29]

Common anxiety disorders[30]

Generalised anxiety disorder (GAD)

GAD involves worrying about a variety of different things, *even when* there is not really anything specific to worry about. This worry is clearly excessive in that it is disproportionate to the actual level of threat. Often a person has trouble sleeping, concentrating, and may be very tense and irritable with others. These issues should be ongoing for at least six months for a diagnosis of GAD to be given.

Post-traumatic stress disorder (PTSD)

This was covered in Chapter 2, 'On Birth'. PTSD can occur when a person has experienced direct trauma or a perceived threat to their health and safety, and then experiences anxiety symptoms as a result. Nightmares, flashbacks and re-experiencing of the trauma might occur, and so might avoidance of things that remind the person of their experience. As an example, someone who experienced birth trauma may avoid sex and/or medical check-ups postpartum, as these things might trigger their anxiety. Other, more general anxiety symptoms are also present, like trouble sleeping, appetite changes, and social withdrawal and isolation. These symptoms need to be present for at least a month following a trauma for a diagnosis of PTSD to be given.

Obsessive compulsive disorder (OCD)

OCD in new mums isn't spoken about often, but I really want to cover it in a bit of depth here, because it is more commonly experienced than we think, given the relative silence on the topic. OCD is the presence of intrusive and unwanted thoughts or images (obsessions) that a person attempts to get rid of or 'neutralise' by performing some other act—also known as a 'compulsion'. When new mothers experience OCD the focus of their unwanted, intrusive thoughts is often the fear of either purposely or accidentally harming their baby. It could also be unwanted sexual thoughts involving their baby. A new mum might have frequent, troubling, irrational—in that they aren't based on any real information or true threat—and intrusive thoughts about her baby getting sick, for instance. She tries to neutralise those thoughts and keep her baby safe by cleaning her hands, again and again and again. A diagnosis of OCD may be given if her compulsive behaviours are excessive—as in, they take up more than an hour of her day on most days, or they have a significant impact on her functioning—as when the compulsion may interfere with her work, social life or mothering.

In some cases, intrusive thoughts are the fear that the mum will *purposely* cause harm, kill, or engage in sexual inappropriateness with her baby. As you can imagine this is incredibly distressing for a new mum. One mum spoke to me about the recurrent, intrusive thought that she was going to throw her baby out of the window or drown her. This is not an uncommon symptom of anxiety and OCD. I want to add here that mums who suffer from this disorder have *absolutely no intention* of harming their babies and aren't considered to be at risk of hurting their babies. In fact, they find it hard to switch off these thoughts because they are about the *very last thing* the mum would *ever* want to do. Her brain is imagining the very worst thing it can think of, and then playing it on repeat, torturing her.

Psychologists often use the following metaphor in anxiety and OCD education and treatment: It's a bit like me telling you right now *not* to think of a red balloon, because if you do it means that you are crazy, and horrible. So it's vital you don't think of that red balloon *right now*. What are you thinking about? Let me guess: a red balloon, right? Mums who suffer intrusive thoughts about hurting their babies find these thoughts disgusting and deplorable, and they try with all their might to stop thinking them. They are so focused on *not* thinking them they can't stop thinking them. All their mental resources are going into *those thoughts*. They will typically engage in 'compulsions' in a subconscious attempt to 'neutralise' the thoughts. This may look like avoidance of physical contact, not being alone with their baby, becoming 'perfectionistic' with cleaning/cooking/routines, excessive checking for signs of harm or other unrelated repetitive actions.

A lot of mums are highly ashamed and afraid to seek help for OCD. They worry that their children will be taken away from them by child protection, or that their partner will feel unsafe leaving them alone with their child. But this is not a child protection issue; it's anxiety. If mums don't tell anyone about these thoughts, they fight them alone, unprotected.

Panic disorder

Panic disorder is when someone experiences panic attacks, and then often worries about having another panic attack. A panic attack can involve trouble breathing, shaking, sweating, fear of dying, dizziness, chest pain, or a feeling of choking, or any combination of these. A person's fear of experiencing another panic attack may cause them to change their normal behaviours to avoid situations they think may trigger them to have another attack. A new mum may begin to isolate herself to avoid having to be around lots of people, for example.

Specific phobia

A specific phobia is when someone has a strong fear of something specific. (I know, you never would have guessed that from the name, right?) People often have fears of spiders, the dark, or heights, for instance. Often when we become mums, our phobia extends to fear for our baby. If someone is afraid of the ocean, they are likely to be very afraid when their baby is around water, and to exaggerate the danger that their baby is in from that specific fear. Walking with a pram on the pier, for example, where there is next to no actual danger, may be a terrifying event for a new mum with a strong, specific fear of the ocean. I know when I attempted my first post-baby pier walk, my legs were like jelly and I could barely place one foot in front of the other.

One common phobia that mums spoke to me about is a sudden, intense fear of dying—fear of getting sick and dying, fear of being in an accident and dying—and no longer being there for their children.

Social phobia

Mums also discussed feeling socially anxious and this worry tended to increase after having their first baby. Lots of women described pathological shyness, and an avoidance of social situations when they became a mum, preferring to isolate themselves at home with their baby. Most mums with social anxiety said that this was because they were afraid of what people were thinking about them and were worried that they would be judged by others. Specifically, a lot of mums were worried that their mothering skills would be being analysed by others.

Common risk factors

A review of the current research has found some common risk factors that are associated with the development of these anxiety disorders. Note that the presence of one or more of these risk factors does not, I repeat, *does not* mean that you are going to develop an anxiety disorder. Similarly, the absence of any of the risk factors does not mean that you won't. These are just things that may make it more likely that a woman will struggle with her anxiety levels in her first year as a mum.

- **Psychological factors:** A mum who has struggled with her mental health in the past may be more likely to experience a recurrence of mental health issues when she first becomes a mum. She may not necessarily have had an anxiety disorder in the past. Her previous mental health history may have included depression, eating disorders, or a personality disorder. Having a low self-esteem has also been associated with poor mental health and anxiety issues for new mums.

- **Demographic factors:** Many studies showed correlations between demographics and prevalence of anxiety among new mums. Mums of a younger age tended to experience anxiety more frequently. Single mums also experienced anxiety more often than partnered mums. Socioeconomic issues, such as having a lower income, having financial or housing worries, and even possessing a Health Care Card, were associated with higher levels of anxiety among new mums.

- **First-time motherhood:** Some studies suggested that first-time mums were at greater risk of developing an anxiety disorder than more experienced mums,[31] but it should be noted that another study told a different story, indicating that mums with more than one child were more anxious than mums of only children.[32]

- **Health and lifestyle:** Mums who smoked or were overweight or obese were also more likely to develop anxiety during their first year postpartum.

- **Genetics and biology:** Having a family history or a biological predisposition to anxiety makes it more likely that a mum will develop an anxiety disorder.

- **Social and relationship issues:** Women with unsupportive partners or an unreliable support network—limited friend or family support—experienced anxiety disorders more often than mums who did have support. Domestic violence was a significant risk factor. Also, women who had experienced a recent 'significant life event'—besides having a baby— were more likely to develop anxiety. Life events may include things like moving house, losing a relative, job loss or relationship changes.

- **Difficulties conceiving or needing intervention to conceive:** Women who have struggled with infertility, took a long time to conceive, mums with previous history of miscarriage or stillbirth, or mums who used IVF to conceive were more prone to anxiety disorders than women who had a more straightforward experience of conception and pregnancy.
- **Baby-specific variables:**[33] A mum's individual and specific experience with her baby had a lot to do with whether she developed an anxiety disorder too. Risk factors include baby being premature, ill, or if they had spent time in the neonatal intensive care unit (NICU). Factors also included difficulties with breastfeeding, sleeping and settling baby.

While more research obviously needs to be done, what is clear is that many women are struggling with anxiety when they become mums. As a society, we need to continue to support research to discover ways to identify women who are at risk of mental health issues during pregnancy or after giving birth. We also need to look out for each other as mums! Everyone is fighting their own battle, and the battle is often invisible.

Her story: Charlotte

When Charlotte gave birth to her first child, she suddenly developed what she described as a 'paranoia-like' fear about death and dying. She said that she was petrified about the everyday, mundane tasks, such as doing errands—she worried she would get into a car crash. She was also terrified of becoming ill and dying. Charlotte said she had a lot of trouble getting off to sleep at night, and that she was often in hysterical tears, worrying about dying.

Charlotte described feeling almost invincible when she was younger and didn't have kids. She felt she had been given an incredible gift and responsibility when she gave birth, and she said that because death is the only way she could imagine not being there for her kids, she became petrified of something happening that was outside of her control. She began to ruminate on what it would be like for her daughter if she had to grow up without a mum.

Charlotte found it helpful to discuss her fears with her husband, in detail, and he gave her great support when she became anxious. She also said that it was helpful when she realised that these things were out of her control and accepted that.

Her story: Sasha

Sasha reported that she had experienced generalised anxiety for most of her life. Then, she had a miscarriage before having her first child two years ago and she experienced bleeding throughout her pregnancy with her now two-year-old. She said that she spent every day of her pregnancy googling stories about miscarriage and bleeding and spotting during pregnancy.

When her son was born, she became extremely anxious about

everything. These thoughts often centred on the health and safety of her baby. She would constantly be on the internet, looking up statistics on sudden infant death syndrome (SIDS), kids' health issues, and major causes of accidents for newborns. She said that she wasn't enjoying her time as a new mother and was incredibly anxious for the time to pass so that her son would be out of the most 'at-risk' time for SIDS and was a bit less vulnerable.

She spent so much of her day worrying about things, that her bonding with her son was being impacted, and her social relationships were impacted too, because of some anxiety around leaving the house—'just in case'. Her anxious thoughts extended to other things too, like having to go back to work, what other people thought about her house, and about her husband's safety when he would be home even five minutes late. She described the first year postpartum as her most creative period, as she was constantly making up elaborate stories in her own mind.

Now that her son is older, she is doing a lot better, but still tends to become anxious and panicky in uncertain situations. She is accessing help from a counsellor concerning these issues, and says she is improving all the time.

Her story: Rachel

Rachel was diagnosed with OCD when she was a teenager. She saw a psychologist at sixteen years of age and learned some good strategies to use when she noticed her intrusive thoughts. These strategies worked well for her, and she was free from OCD symptoms for about five years before she fell pregnant with her first son.

When he was born, Rachel noticed intrusive thoughts almost immediately, but now they were mostly focused on her son. When she gave her son a bath, the image of her pushing him underwater and drowning him wouldn't leave her mind. When she tried to settle him at night, the image of throwing him out of the window replayed. She began to find ways to avoid being alone with her son in what she saw as compromising situations. She would ask her husband to bathe him and would purposely (but seemingly accidentally) wake him up when the baby cried at night.

She didn't tell her husband about these thoughts, and these behaviours started to impact on their relationship. She said she was afraid that he would think she was crazy, and that he wouldn't trust her with their son, ever. She was even afraid that he might call child protection services. Some days she wondered if she should call them herself. Eventually, she did explain everything to him, and sought some help from a psychologist. She knew there were strategies that had worked for her in the past, but she needed a refresher on them. Her psychologist also referred her to a psychiatrist, who prescribed some medication.

She is going well now, but she suffered alone for a long time before seeking support, and she regrets this now.

Let's get practical

As discussed, both our limbic system and our prefrontal cortex can't be in control of us at the same time. Our limbic system handles our emotions, while our prefrontal cortex is our brain's rational, logic centre. When anxiety is triggered, our limbic system is the boss. We need to find a way to calm that system and to hand over system control to our prefrontal cortex, before we will manage to respond logically to a situation, before we will manage our anxiety. But how?

Similar to the depression treatment discussed in the last chapter, we struggle to manage our unhelpful thoughts until we begin to manage our physiological symptoms—managing these will put us in a better headspace to both recognise, and challenge, unhelpful thoughts.

Never was the need for first-line, practical, anxiety-management strategies more evident to me than while I was lying prostrate in an MRI machine. As you know, I tend towards anxiety and this day was no exception. I wasn't thrilled about the prospect of being stuck inside a small tube for an hour plus. After lots of practice, I'm usually very good at managing my anxiety levels when they spike. But on this day, my good-old first-line strategies were suddenly not available to me!

I was having an MRI on my entire spine. The technician had asked me to lie *completely still* to allow the machine to take clear pictures of my neck and back. After the first round of pictures, the MRI technician told me to 'relax'. The pictures were too blurry. I was breathing too deeply and it was making my head move too much. Slow, controlled breathing is the way that I usually slow my heart rate, and thus, slow down the release of stress hormones and the resulting physiological changes discussed before. If it's too late for that, another strategy I use to 'burn off' the energy caused by the stress hormones is to move around—shake, tense and release my muscles, exercise. For obvious reasons, this was not an option either. All of my usual tricks were out of the question in that damn tube!

I began to breathe more shallowly, attempting to stay still, but this increased my anxiety levels and I was *too* tense. I began hyperventilating and swallowing a lot and the MRI technician was unable to get the required pictures. Eventually he stopped the scan without finishing and asked me to consider sedative medication next time. This was just slightly humbling, for someone who makes a living helping other people manage their anxiety.

My point is that the technician told me several times throughout the scan to 'relax'. He told me to 'calm down', and that 'nothing bad will happen'. I knew that, logically. Isn't this our constant inner dialogue? Don't we tell ourselves this all the time while we are experiencing anxiety? But our logical brain is not in control in that moment. Our emotional brain is. So we aren't going to be able to fight against ourselves, until we hand over that control and calm our emotional brain. I, a clinical psychologist with over fifteen years' experience in learning about and teaching anxiety management techniques to other people, could not manage my anxiety without my seemingly simple, first-line behavioural strategies. It's impossible to manage by our own wishes and will. It's not the way our brains and bodies are designed.

Behavioural strategies for anxiety management

Like I said, similar to depression treatment, we need to make behavioural changes before we will be able to make any cognitive changes needed to manage anxiety. As I noticed in the MRI machine, my brain was in no condition to calm down, or 'not worry about it' while my limbic system was running hot and taking the lead. There are some first-line behavioural changes we can make in order to set ourselves up for a more successful journey to healing from anxiety. Then, when we are better at recognising our anxiety signs, managing our anxiety from a physiological point of view, and handing over system control to our rational brains, we can begin to challenge our unhelpful anxious cognitions, or thoughts.

As mentioned before, the strategies discussed here are a start, but are not meant to take the place of a personalised mental health treatment plan. Please seek additional help if you feel you need some support around any anxiety issue. Your GP is a great place to begin that journey.

Recognise your anxiety signs

Every person is unique so not everyone's anxiety presents the same way. We need to begin by observing our own feelings and behaviour, in order to become experts on our own mental health. Biologically and psychologically, the earlier we begin intervening in our body's anxiety response the better, so recognition of our earliest anxiety signs is crucial.

Begin by taking notes in your journal after an episode of anxiety. Think back to what was going on directly before that episode, how you felt and what you did. After a while, you will begin to see patterns that will show you your own earliest anxiety signs. Some common early signs are:

- hypervigilance
- feelings of dread or apprehension
- feeling jumpy
- feeling 'blank' like your mind is empty or having trouble concentrating
- heart racing
- headaches
- muscle tension
- tummy upset
- sweatiness
- trouble breathing
- irritability
- shaking.

Once we are familiar with our own early anxiety signs, we can begin to apply our first-line behavioural strategies at the earliest possible stage.

Deep breathing

During episodes of anxiety, our hearts are racing, so they pump around hormones such as adrenaline, which gives us energy to run or fight from threats, and cortisol, a stress hormone, much faster than they would otherwise. We don't want this, unless we are faced with an actual threat, like an attacker. Otherwise, there's not much use for these hormones and nowhere for them to escape to, and they remain in our body causing us harm and chronic health issues over time.

We can slow our heart rates—and subsequently these hormones rushing through our body—by slowing down our breathing. Take some slow, deep breaths—in through your nose, and out through your mouth—as soon as you notice your early anxiety signs. Try to keep that heart rate as regular as possible. A good technique to try is 'triangle breathing': in through your nose for three seconds, hold for three seconds, out through your mouth for three seconds. Put one hand on your tummy and one on your chest. The hand on your tummy should go in as you breathe in, and out as you breathe out.

Regular practice of slow, controlled, deep breathing will help maintain a lower cortisol level, and will also make it more likely that you will remember to breathe when your anxiety is next triggered.

Dive reflex

We humans come equipped with something called the mammalian diving response. This is an automatic reflex that kicks in when we are submerged in cold water, or even when we do something like splash cold water on our face. The trigeminal nerves all over our face detect that we might be about to take a swim, and they send out a message to our vagus nerve, which connects our brain with our body, to tell our body to slow down our heart rates, preparing us for an underwater environment. As we know, a slow heart rate equals slowing the fight or flight response, so this is a cool (literally), quick anxiety-management trick. It just requires a quick trip to the nearest sink.

Move

Like we discussed, once our fight or flight response has switched on, our body is in survival mode. We need to find a way to burn off the excess energy caused by the rush of stress hormones that have flooded our body, preparing us to fight or flee. In an actual emergency we would do this naturally by fighting the threat or running away from it. In a perceived emergency, we need to be creative.

Depending on your situation, where you are and the time you have available, this might look like a full workout or run, shaking your body, or dancing around your lounge room. If you are out and about, you might remove yourself from a situation and go for a brisk walk around the block. Even five minutes of exercise can begin to give us anti-anxiety effects. As well as burning off stress hormones, the way our body is designed, exercise also increases endorphins, which are a natural antidote to cortisol. Exercise also helps us relax more fully, and to sleep more deeply.

Grounding

Grounding techniques guide a person to remain in the present moment, instead of being stuck in the past (ruminating) or the future (worrying), which is so common for anxious people. They help us to focus on the here and now, using our five basic senses: hearing, smell, touch, taste and sight. This helps us to feel in control of our realities and emotions. A popular grounding activity is the 5-4-3-2-1 Grounding Technique, which is included at the end of this section. I do this myself each night before bed.

It really helps to hand back control to that rational part of the brain, the prefrontal cortex.

Cognitive techniques
Unhelpful thinking habits—anxiety

Now that our rational brain, our prefrontal cortex, is switched on and in control, we can begin to apply strategies to assist us with our unhelpful cognitions, or thinking habits. If you suffer from anxiety, you are likely to be having a lot of unhelpful, anxiety-laden thoughts on a day-to-day basis. These are hard to shift, as your brain and body are working to protect you. Letting go of your anxious thoughts is asking you to let go of some of your armour. Our goal is to let them take a bit of a break; they are working overtime right now.

Unhelpful thinking habits were discussed in Chapter 8, 'On Postpartum Depression', so I'm just going to provide here a few basic examples of common *anxiety-related* unhelpful cognitions, but feel free to review the section in the depression chapter to refresh your memory as well. Examples of anxious unhelpful thinking habits are:

- **Jumping to conclusions:** When we jump to conclusions, we predict the future based on little (or no) evidence. A new mum, for example, chooses not to attend her local community mothers' group because she assumes (with no evidence) that everyone there will know more about being a mum than she does, and that they will all notice that she doesn't know what she is doing.

- **Catastrophising:** When we catastrophise, we blow things out of proportion. For example, a new mum who needs to go back to work in a few months may spend a lot of her maternity leave time excessively worrying about potential negative effects that she worries this could have on her baby.
- **Shoulding and musting:** Should thoughts and must thoughts place unreasonable pressure on us. A new mum having trouble with her breast milk supply, for instance, may feel extremely upset, like she is failing as a mum, because she believes she *must* breastfeed for her baby to be healthy.
- **Emotional reasoning:** Emotional reasoning is where we believe that if we *feel* a certain way then something *is* a certain way. We assume our automatic feelings are always a reflection of reality. Say we feel anxious about some aspects of parenthood, then we think this is a sign that we have no idea what we are doing and that we are bad parents.
- **Overgeneralising:** This occurs when we make assumptions and predictions about the future based on limited evidence. We think that if something happens once, it is likely to happen again. Consider the new mum with a squirmy new baby who slipped out of her arms in the bath one time, and his face briefly went underwater. She pulled him out after less than a second, but she becomes excessively anxious around bath time and begins to believe that she is not capable of bathing the baby by herself.

Our unhelpful thinking habits usually aren't accurate. However, they are hard to break because they are part of such an automatic, often long-term pattern of thinking that we likely aren't even aware of their existence. Often these thoughts are based on our core beliefs too. Remember core beliefs are often present from as early as childhood, and serve to form our views of ourselves, others and the world. It's extremely tough to work through these beliefs, and I recommend a personal therapist for assistance in doing so.

We must be strategic about *how* and *when* we begin to focus on and challenge these unhelpful thinking habits. The danger is, by giving them airtime and focusing on them more, we water these seeds, and strengthen the roads (neural pathways) associated with them. Remember the red balloon example? We don't want all our cognitive energy going into these thoughts. But we also don't want to leave them to be. So what to do?

As I noted in the MRI machine, and as you would have noticed when you tried not to think of red balloons before (you're still doing it, aren't you?), we can't just tell ourselves not to worry anymore. If we try to push away and stop the thoughts we automatically have, we focus our attention and energy on them even more. We are watering and growing those seeds. We need to *retrain* our brains by being very deliberate about how and when—and when not—to focus on our unhelpful thoughts and challenge our unhelpful cognitions.

Worry time

I suggest *postponing* your worry. Many people benefit from designating a specific 'worry time' to their day. Instead of giving airtime to your worries every time they appear, giving them your time and energy and strengthening them, and rather than ignoring or suppressing them, letting them eat you up alive, postpone them. You can retrain your brain to realise that you don't need to answer the door each time anxiety comes knocking. This postponing provides us with a time to worry, problem-solve and to talk, but also allows us not to live our life dominated by anxious thoughts, or to make them stronger by focusing on them all the time.

A designated worry time is most helpful when allocated for a similar time each day. This trains our brain to naturally postpone worry during the rest of the day. Choose a morning or early afternoon worry time if your schedule allows it. We don't want you to go to sleep thinking about your worries. A worry time should be no longer than half an hour, but always, *always*, cut it short and get on with your day, if you find you are running out of things to worry about! Set a timer and be strict with yourself about not going over it. You can always worry more again tomorrow! Plan something nice for after your worry time—a chat with a positive friend, a cup of herbal tea or a walk—to help you ease back into the rest of your day.

By now, you are probably wondering what one *does* during a designated worry time? Well, first we need to determine whether the things we are worrying about are solvable or unsolvable. Remember the Serenity Prayer that was on everyone's nanna's toilet door when they were little: *'God, grant me the serenity to accept the things I cannot change, / Courage to change the things I can, / And wisdom to know the difference.'* If a worry is solvable, then we can use our worry time to *problem-solve* it.

Think about and write down the problem. Brainstorm all the ways you can think of to solve the problem. No solution is too silly, impossible, outlandish or illegal. (For this activity—there are definitely things that are too illegal in real life!) Once you've got a list of possible solutions, choose a few favourites and consider what you think would happen if you apply these solutions. Which option sounds best? That's what you'll try. If that doesn't go well, you can repeat the activity tomorrow. For now, you've got a plan; that worry can rest for now.

You can also use your worry time to *talk* to someone about your worries if you choose to. Talking about your worries with a trusted, non-judgemental person is one of the best ways to diffuse anxious thoughts and feelings. Talking makes anxious thoughts less scary. By running them past a screener we test their accuracy and likelihood, and by saying them out loud, we put them in a more realistic perspective. Most of the time our worries are groundless, and talking about them out loud can help us to see that. In other cases where worries are warranted, talking allows us to bounce our problem-solving ideas off someone and benefit from their outsider perspective and unbiased experience.

We can also use our worry time to *challenge* our unhelpful thinking patterns. The 'You be the judge' activity from the depression chapter (Chapter 8) and the table will be of help here.

The Thought	
Evidence FOR the Thought	**Evidence AGAINST the Thought**
The Verdict	

During your designated worry time, create a table in your journal and write down all the evidence that you have *for* the thoughts and worries that you are having and, more importantly, all of the evidence you have *against* them. Remember, evidence includes cold-hard facts only. No opinions, guesses or assumptions are allowed during this activity. Based on your work, ask yourself the following questions:

- Are these thoughts true?
- How likely are these things to happen?
- What are some more likely outcomes?
- What is the worst that could happen if these things were to happen?
- What would *you tell someone else who was worrying about these things?*

In reality, some of our worries *will* actually be warranted; as in, things that actually are likely to cause an issue. Financial pressures or family health issues are some examples. If our worries are warranted, then have a go at problem-solving them, and also ask yourself the following questions:

- Is this helpful for me to think about right now?
- Is this solvable or not?
- What would I tell a friend in a similar situation? Does the same advice apply to me? Can I be as gentle with myself as I would with them?
- Who can help me through this?

Outside of your worry time, you can make notes of the feelings, thoughts and worries that come to your mind, but you are making a mental agreement with yourself *not* to go into them until later. The notes are merely to remind you of your worries in order to focus on them in your worry time. A lot of the time you will find that your notes impact you less after you've postponed your worries; a result of the brain being gradually retrained.

It's so easy to set aside time to concentrate on this stuff with all the extra time you have on maternity leave with a newborn baby isn't it? (Insert massive eye-roll here.) Sorry about that. I know these things take a lot of work and energy. I've only recently been in your new-mum shoes and some days I barely had time to wash my face, let alone change my brain structure. With some careful planning and discussion with your support team, I do believe it is do-able though, and well worth it in the end. Don't beat yourself up (at all!) if you don't get to do these techniques 'perfectly'—whatever that means. Every time you try something, you make a difference, and you are gradually healing yourself. This will have a snowball effect for you; each change elicits more significant change. You can get there.

Outside of worry time, during the rest of your day, you must train your brain to postpone worry, with the goal of ultimately resetting some of your hard-wired anxious neural pathways. Work on ways to enjoy your life, worry less, and be in the present moment with your beautiful new baby.

Strategies for postponing worry

Many of us think of relaxation time as watching TV or scrolling social media with coffee and chocolate. Though these things are nice, we need to practise specific relaxation techniques to train our brains long-term, strengthen our prefrontal cortex, calm our limbic system and help with the connection between the two, so that they work as a team.

Regular practice of targeted relaxation strategies can physically train the brain to worry less, not just feel relaxed in the moment, like with watching TV where no lasting positive change is taking place.

Mindfulness meditation

Mindfulness is the ability to be fully present, and live 'in the moment'. Regular practice of mindfulness meditation increases our ability to regulate our own anxiety levels. It teaches us to accept our constant stream of anxious thoughts for what they are, without judging them, and then to turn our attention towards something else more positive and meaningful. Outside of our worry time, this is what we are working to achieve—leaning away from anxiety, rather than into it.

Regular, intentional practice of mindfulness meditation is a good way to train our brain to focus on what we *do* want, rather than what we *don't* want. As we practise it intentionally, we learn this skill on such a deep level that it begins to happen automatically, by default, in our everyday lives. We become more present in the here and now.

There are many, many, many aps to help you with mindfulness meditation if you choose to use them. It is very simple though, so all you really need is yourself.

Choose a comfortable place to sit, with as little distraction as possible. Choose an amount of time you want to meditate for—at first, this might only be five minutes, then it will likely get longer over time. Set a timer so that you don't spend the whole time obsessing about when you are going to finish and clock watching. Now spend a few minutes sitting quietly and breathing and begin to focus on your breath and the sensations in your body. Use your breath as your anchor to ground yourself in the present moment. Turn your attention towards how it feels to breathe in and then out. Your attention will wander away from your breathing—probably lots of times. This is okay. It is your job to notice when this happens—it doesn't matter if it takes you a while to notice—and to gently and non-judgementally draw your attention back to the feeling of breathing. Come back to your breathing as many times as it takes, until your timer goes off.

That's it! That's all you do.

This practice teaches your brain that it doesn't need to engage with each thought that enters it. With time and practice, this will become more automatic.

When I first learned this technique in my first year at university, I was taught using a sultana. Instead of breathing, we were asked to focus on the sensory experience of the sultana in our mouths—how it felt, how it tasted, how it smelled. This is a good technique if you prefer something external to you to help you stay focused. My second-year teacher, however, taught the same lesson using a packet of Rolos. For some strange reason, her lectures were always more popular!

Mindfulness in everyday life

Let's be realistic. As a new mum, some days, you will *not* have time to meditate. Some days the thought of setting aside fifteen minutes for a mindfulness session will seem akin to climbing Mount Everest. (That's what I call my laundry pile.) When you just don't have the time, the good news is that you can incorporate mindfulness practice into your everyday life. A shower, washing dishes, eating, rhythmic exercise—as in walking, jogging or swimming, nothing you need to concentrate too hard on—can all be done mindfully. This way, you are not using any extra time, and you are sneaking into your day some brain training. The key is to focus on your sensory experience. If you are showering, you will be focusing on the feel of the water, the smell of the shampoo, and the sounds of water rushing. You will be drawing your attention back to that sensory experience, when it wanders off into anxiety territory.

It's good to note that when we get anxious we tend to seek out and grasp onto our anxiety triggers. Our brains are trying to protect us, and we hold fast to our protector. So, we find ourselves up at all hours of the night browsing horror stories of babies left in car seats, strange symptoms that develop into deadly illnesses, or kidnappings, as if the more we focus on them the less likely they will be to happen to us. We might google our own and our baby's symptoms until we find the most serious possible cause for that rash or lump and then we obsess over it. Instead of leaning into our anxiety in this way, we need to try to lean away from it. Try to identify what is triggering your anxiety, and lean away, rather than towards it. I'm not talking about avoidance of life, or the things we have to do, but I am talking about not going out of your way to seek out anxiety.

Behavioural experiment—exposure

Avoidance increases anxiety. The socially anxious person who begins to avoid social functions out of fear of judgement becomes even more socially anxious, and subsequently more socially avoidant. It's a vicious, unrelenting cycle.

The key to overcoming anxiety for good is to face it. Confront it gradually, in small steps—as small as you need. I really suggest working with a professional psychologist to make your plan around this gradual exposure to your fear. If you try to do it alone, you risk making it worse. Your psychologist will work with you to break down your fear into tiny steps, ranging from what scares you least to what scares you most, and will help and encourage you to safely, gradually face your fears—with the help of the behavioural and cognitive strategies we've been talking about of course.

Enlist partner support

Enlisting the support of your partner, if you have one, has consistently been found to be an important part of anxiety treatment.[34] It has been found to be effective to talk about the specifics of your anxiety and specific fears, like in Charlotte's story. If you don't have a partner, or don't feel comfortable talking to them, enlist the support of a friend or family member who you do feel comfortable talking with.

5-4-3-2-1 grounding exercise

This exercise aims to give you control over your own reality and emotions. Take a few slow, deep, triangle breaths to focus. We are aiming to ground you and bring you into the present moment.

Look around: What are *5* things that you can see? The couch, the oven, your baby? Say them out loud.

Feel: What are *4* things that you can feel right now? Your cosy socks, your baby's breath, a breeze on your neck? Say them out loud.

Listen: Listen out for *3* things that you can hear. Do you hear traffic outside, music playing, your baby babbling? Say these things out loud.

Smell: What are *2* things that you can smell? Coffee brewing, a candle, your baby's head? (If you can't smell anything, name your two favourite smells.) Say them out loud.

Taste: What's the *1* thing you taste right now? (If you can't taste anything, think of your favourite thing to taste.) Say it out loud.

Reflection

- Have you noticed yourself becoming any more anxious since becoming a mum? What types of things trigger your anxiety?
- What do you think some of your early anxiety signs are?
- Did you recognise any of the unhelpful thinking habits in your own patterns of thinking?
- Are there any barriers to incorporating some of the anxiety management strategies (like worry time or mindfulness meditation) into your day? Time, space, support? What are some ways to overcome these barriers?
- Have you spoken to anyone about your worries, and if not, who might be a good person to talk to?

10

On Relationships:
The best of times,
the worst of times

So, you've just had a baby. Now, get ready to meet your baby's other parent. That's right! You are about to meet your co-parent. Yes, you already know each other but you are about to see your partner in a whole new light. You both have brand new roles to play. You have never parented together before, and this could get interesting!

People say that the first year postpartum is the hardest on relationships. You are about to see your partner's most endearing and their most infuriating qualities, sometimes both in the space of one hour. Having a baby can be both the best and the worst thing to happen to a relationship. *At the same time!*

Your partner will astonish you with their tenderness, baffle you with their logic—or lack thereof—delight you with their humour, amaze you with their capacity for love, madden you with their priorities and exasperate you with their very presence.

Watching my husband become a dad was one of the greatest moments I have ever experienced. I saw that he was enamoured from the first moment he laid eyes on our son. (Well, not the *first* moment—I didn't witness that, as I steadfastly refused to look down at the war zone going on whence our son emerged.) Still now, over three years later, we can be found looking at each other, wonder in our eyes, and gushing, 'How on earth did *we* make *him*?'

As I've already described, it took a while for me to warm up to becoming a mum. My husband, though, took to parenthood like a duck to water. When our son napped, and I felt complete and utter freedom, he said he missed him. *Missed him*! Can you believe it?! He was even known to ask if he could wake him up after he had been asleep for a mere fifteen minutes. (Why no, sir. That would be a negatory.)

Sometimes—okay, a lot—this stark contrast between our ease of adjustment to parenting was a source of distress for me. Even though I was thrilled to see them bonding, and to see how much they clearly adored each other, I sometimes wondered why I didn't feel like that. I could safely say that I had *never* missed our son during nap time—never! I love him so much, but last week I told him that he needed to nap because 'we need some time apart from each other'.

On some particularly bad days, I illogically thought my husband was doing it on purpose to rub it in my face. Every time he was an awesome parent and did awesome parent things, it felt like a personal attack and it highlighted my own incompetence.

I felt like I was crawling to the finish line each day, while he was sprinting laps around me. Who was this person? Why was he beating me at this?

I realised early on that it is useless to compare ourselves with other parents—*including our own partners!* We all have different temperaments, personality types, lives, histories and needs.

The transition to parenthood can be the most amazing life change for a couple. You suddenly see the person you love in a whole new role, in a whole new light, in a whole new relationship. It's truly amazing to see a person form a relationship with their child, and even more so when they're also your child. How beautiful is that?

It can also be very challenging. Your family dynamic has changed. Once you were two people, now you are three—or more if you have twins or triplets! You might be very accustomed to your life as a twosome. I know we were. As I've said before, we were together a long time before our son was born and had a cosy, predictable life that was *all about us*. On top of this change in dynamic you are hormonal, sleep-deprived, bone-weary, crazy-busy, and have a tiny person to look after 24/7. This mental-load on both of you can be an explosive cocktail of conflict and resentment waiting to happen.

A 2000 study found that 67 per cent of postpartum couples experienced a decrease in marital satisfaction after becoming parents for the first time.[35] It makes sense. The adjustment to new parenthood is massive, and there are a lot of factors that understandably contribute to conflict and an overall decrease in relationship satisfaction. Exhaustion, time-pressure, worry and anxiety, financial pressure—perhaps going down to one income—and focus on the new baby instead of each other can combine with disastrous results for couples. The same study found that factors that buffered against this outcome were the quality of the couple's friendship *before* the baby came along, continued fondness for and admiration of each other, and the continued focus on and awareness of the relationship. Also, maintaining a sense of teamwork and unity was important in maintaining relationship satisfaction in the postpartum period. We need to remember that we are on the same team!

It's okay that couples fight. The most solid and happy couples in the world fight. They can even go through periods where one or both partners are unsatisfied in the relationship. What's important is that couples 'fight right' and utilise good communication skills when disagreeing or going through tough periods in the relationship. There are some common problems I came across when talking to new mums about their relationships postpartum.

Comparing and competing

I believe this is one of the most important lessons to learn when a couple become parents for the first time. As humans, we tend to compare, compete and keep track. It's a toxic environment to live in when a couple is constantly competing—from who changed the last nappy to who woke up the most times last night and who is the most tired. There is *always* something to compete over. The problem is, when we spend time doing this we invite a number of complications into our lives.

We continuously focus on the negatives of our partners, for one thing. Like that seed, what we water—focus on—grows. If we are concentrating all day on what our partner *didn't* do, and how they are lacking, then that is what we will notice more of. Resentment grows and a toxic environment begins to form. Instead, water gratitude. Try to focus on what your partner did. Try to focus less on comparing and more on teamwork.

Lack of effective communication

Have you ever said one thing, but felt like the person you were talking to heard something completely different? Like you were speaking English, but they were listening in binary code? Sometimes people, even couples that have been together for years, have such completely different ways of communicating that they often fail to pick up what the other person is laying out for them. This could be for several reasons.

Sometimes we think we know what someone is going to say, so we mentally fill in the blanks without truly listening to their words. We spend the time they are speaking planning an argument in our head instead of listening to what they say. Lots of pointless miscommunications and disagreements happen that way. Sometimes sleep deprivation, anxiety or the baby blues make us impatient, snappy and less communicative. Sometimes couples are poor communicators in general. It's never too late to learn communication skills and they can be amazingly effective in helping couples to navigate parenthood as a team.

Psychologist Dr John Gottman has been researching relationships for decades upon decades. Over several studies, he has shown that he can predict the eventual success/failure rate of a couple with 91 per cent accuracy, just by watching and listening to them communicate with each other for as little as five minutes![36] For obvious reasons (91 per cent accuracy, you guys!) he is considered an authority on communication. He says that fighting and arguing are not a problem within a partnership; rather, it is *the way we argue,* the way we communicate with each other through adversity—that is what matters. In his book *The Seven Principles for Making Marriage Work*, Gottman outlined some of the signs that indicate a couple is heading down a dangerous path, communication-wise, and the things he warns us to look out for include the way we begin conversations, the way we treat each other during interactions, and how we regulate our own emotions during arguments, among other things.

Poor communication is not uncommon but it's never too late to change the way we communicate with each other. I strongly recommend both partners read Gottman's book to learn more about effective (and ineffective) communication—and see if you can improve on the way you communicate with and treat each other; especially during the highly sensitive and already vulnerable transition into new parenthood.

Seeing each other as parents—and nothing else

You've become parents, and are in this bubble of newness, of transition and of responsibility. Okay, but you are still *you*. Your partner is still who they are, too. You both still individually have thoughts, values, passions, needs and wants *outside* of being a mum or a dad. Sometimes we can forget that. Not only for ourselves but for our partners. We can begin to look at them like our relay race partner, so eager to pass them the baton of parenthood for a minute so we can go pee, or sleep, or eat, that we are like passing ships in the night. We stop *seeing* each other—at least seeing each other outside of a teammate, a co-parent, or an extra hand.

You need to prioritise time to be together, and to talk about things other than your baby. Yes, you love the baby, and yes they need a lot of discussion and attention right now, but your relationship was the beginning of their life. It will be one of the most important foundational aspects of their development as they grow. Your relationship is so important that it's functioning can actually impact on your baby's growth and development.[37] For your own sake and your baby's, your relationship needs to be one of your top priorities during this tough transition period. You really need to have quality time together. I know, I know, it is *way* easier said than done when you barely have time to pee alone. Manageable ways to prioritise your relationship will be discussed in the 'Let's Get Practical' section below.

Lack of support

I'm talking here about actual lack of support and not the perceived lack of support that can come from comparing and competing for every nappy change and wake up in the night. If one partner is not pulling their weight, it places an incredible burden on the other. Reasons for this disparity can be many and varied: anxiety, depression, sleep deprivation, uncertainty, busy-ness, cultural expectations—for example, the thought that a woman is responsible for the baby and the home, or a man must be the breadwinner. It is more than okay to give ourselves a break during the postpartum period, but this becomes a problem if one person is doing all of the work that has to be accomplished. If one person is carrying the physical—feeding the baby, changing the baby, settling the baby, cooking, paying bills, earning money, and the housework—and mental load, this can cause enormous resentment and distress. Most people have individual strengths, skills and talents, so you may like to split up required tasks in advance, depending on what you like to do—or dislike the least, perhaps.

Not looking out for one another

So many people struggle to look after themselves. We fail to prioritise our own health, let alone our own happiness. If we are in a partnership, not only do we need to look out for our baby and ourselves, we also need to look out for one another. We need to prioritise each other's health, well-being and happiness. We should be on the lookout for signs that our partner is struggling and needs us to step in, or ways that we can make their day sunnier, or their night more relaxing. Research shows that one of the keys to happiness is to focus on what we can do for others.[38] Who better to focus on making happy than our partner? An added bonus to this is, while we are focusing on what we can do to make our partner's life better, they can focus on us right back. Win–win!

Mirroring each other

Have you ever found yourself in a perfectly fine mood, only to have your partner arrive home in a stinker? You then suddenly feel angry, frustrated and on-edge for no reason? This could be mirror neurons at work. Mirror neurons, a relatively recent discovery, are predicted to transform the field of neuroscience. Mirror neurons cause our brains to pretend that we experience what we observe—to 'mirror' the experience of others. This can be a good thing, as it helps us connect to and empathise with others.

We are social creatures, and our brains are wired to connect with others. However, when one person in a partnership is frustrated, stressed or anxious—which happens a lot in early parenthood—the other can be easily influenced by that. This means that for our own and our partner's benefits, we need to be proactive about our postpartum emotional regulation and mental health.

Sexual relationship, or lack thereof

It is not uncommon for women to experience a lack of desire for, and enjoyment in, sex postpartum. A 2016 study found that both mental and physical enjoyment of and satisfaction in sex was lower postpartum than before pregnancy.[39] It also found that only 43 per cent of women had resumed intercourse by week six postpartum, which went up to 92 per cent at twelve weeks postpartum. If you don't feel ready or are not enjoying things the way you think you 'should', rest assured, you are not alone.

This lack of satisfaction may last for several weeks or even up to a year for many women. There are lots of reasons. When we first bring baby home, lots of us are dealing with ceasarean or episiotomy wounds, vaginal tears and stitches. The thought of anyone coming near us, particularly in an intimate way, can be traumatising, especially if we've had a difficult birth. Long-term sexual function is unlikely to be impacted but vaginal pain and sexual discomfort is a common experience for at least a few months postpartum.[40] When we try to 'push past the pain' or engage in sex when we aren't ready, this can make matters worse, causing pain and increasing our anxiety around sex and intimacy.

New mums can also feel 'touched out'. They often spend their days holding, rocking and feeding baby, and when baby is finally asleep, more touching is often last on their list of priorities. Fatigue, stress and body confidence also have their parts to play in the lack of sexual drive for many women.

One Australian study found that 16 per cent of women didn't

want to have sex during their first year of motherhood, while 7 per cent didn't enjoy it when they did have sex.[41] Reasons for the lack of desire included tiredness and lack of energy, irritability and tension; whereas lack of enjoyment tended to be caused by relationship issues, like not feeling supported by a partner, or frequent disagreements in the home. This study focused on adoptive as well as biological mothers, so the results clearly weren't caused just by the birthing process.

Women who struggle with the adjustment to parenthood, and women who experience mental health issues postpartum are most likely to be affected by a lack of sexual desire and enjoyment. So, if you are experiencing any of these issues around postpartum sex, you are certainly not alone! These feelings will most likely resolve themselves in time. We need to be patient with our bodies— they have just accomplished quite a feat! Your body will feel like yours again.

Their story: Michelle and Tony

Michelle and Tony had been in a relationship for five years— married for two—before having their daughter Lilly. When Lilly was two weeks old, Michelle said that one day, while she was feeding Lilly her bottle, she looked over at Tony, who was making a coffee in the kitchen, and she thought 'I miss that man'. She felt ridiculous, because he hadn't gone anywhere; in fact, they had been spending more time together than ever before. He hadn't returned to work after his paternity leave yet, and they were up together all hours of the day and night. But she felt like they hadn't been 'themselves' or spoken about anything other than Lilly since she was born.

What she missed were their simple connections that she said she had taken for granted. Their freedom to 'just be together' watching a movie on the couch, to spontaneously decide to go out for a meal, to talk about whatever they wanted, whenever they wanted, without interruption, to fall asleep in each other's arms, for an uninterrupted night. She said she couldn't remember the last time they had cuddled, or even gone to bed at the same time.

She felt silly saying anything to Tony but one day she started crying and couldn't stop. She told him how she'd been feeling and, to her surprise, he said he'd been feeling the same way. He said he hadn't wanted to say anything to her, as she seemed so focused on Lilly and he didn't want to add to her stress or make her feel that she had to worry about him, too. Together, they devised ways they could 'keep the spark alive'. Lilly was quite a good sleeper in her pram, so they discovered they could still go out for breakfast or lunch, or a long walk, and have an uninterrupted hour of together time. They started making the effort to talk about things other than parenting. They found their connection beginning to deepen as they focused on their relationship, and they started to feel 'more in love than ever before'.

Their story: Nora and Jimmy

Nora said that she and her partner Jimmy had never had a fight before they became parents. Never! When their son came along, they couldn't *stop* fighting. Nora said she felt like she 'hated'

Jimmy. She used to seethe with anger when he left a dish in the sink or went to take a nap. She swore at him under her breath every time he left the room. She said that everything about him began to annoy her. She didn't speak to anyone about this; she thought she was the only one secretly hating her partner, as when she looked around, all she could see were happy couples!

Nora eventually figured out that her anger was frustration at the discrepancies between their life changes. Jimmy still went to work, got a full night's sleep, and went to the gym. Nora stayed at home with the baby and was the one getting up at night to feed him. She didn't have any time to herself. Nora's whole life had changed. The baby was now her whole life; for Jimmy, she felt, the baby was a nice addition, but didn't change anything for him.

When Nora figured this out, she thought she'd better discuss this with him. When she did, she found that he had been feeling the discrepancy, too. Only he thought that Nora was leaving him out of things and did not want his help. He thought that she saw him as useless with the baby, and that he was hoping to have more parental responsibilities when he became a dad. He felt left out and useless. He felt angry towards Nora. Each of them felt anger towards the other, but no one was talking about it. After they had shared their perspectives, things became a lot smoother around the house. Sharing the load helped each of them feel respected and heard.

Their story: Sara and Todd

Sara had an episiotomy when she gave birth to her son. After the birth, this caused her a lot of pain for a long time, and she felt anxious about the thought of sex. She was in a mothers' group and when, at around the six-week postpartum mark, other new mums started talking about having sex, she was floored. Other people were having sex already? She thought the idea sounded terrifying. She wasn't ready. But she thought she must have been the only one not having sex, so she felt guilty.

She made up reasons not to have sex with her husband, Todd, who began to feel rejected. He didn't push, but Sara knew that he was questioning her desire for him. She felt absolutely no desire for sex, but it wasn't to do with Todd. She had no drive. At around twelve weeks postpartum Sara and Todd did have sex, and she was surprised that it didn't hurt as much as she thought it would and that physically things were essentially back to normal. She stopped feeling anxious about sex. But she still doesn't feel much of a drive.

Her son is one now, and things haven't really gotten back to normal in that way. Sara is in love with Todd, they are happy, but sex is not as much a part of their lives as it once was. She knows this can be normal for some women and hopes that her drive will return soon. In the meantime, Sara and Todd are doing their best to communicate well, to spend quality time together and to show each other love in lots of different ways.

Let's get practical

Here are some ideas for keeping your relationship happy and healthy after baby arrives.

Quality time

Time is a precious commodity when you are new parents! When you finally get time to yourself, your brain overloads on 'What do I do: Shower, sleep, eat, watch TV?' There is so much to do in so little child-free time. Often your relationship takes a backseat to your *freedom*! However, as we discussed above, our relationship does need to be a priority at this time, to keep it healthy, alive and growing. Some ideas for making quality time a reality are:

- **Date nights in:** It may not be possible to—or you may not want to—get someone to look after baby while you go out on a date night. But during one of your baby's naps, you might like to have a date night in. Watch a good movie, play cards, or break out the chessboard. Or just talk and connect. Make a picnic and have it on the floor. Have a candlelit takeaway dinner, or a tub of ice cream to share. Talk about things other than the baby. Have sex, if you want. Connect and remember you were a couple first, before you were parents. You will be a couple long after your kids move out. Prioritise each other.
- **Bring baby on a date:** Many young babies are reasonable sleepers in their pram. If you are one of these lucky parents, consider going on a brunch, lunch or dinner date with your baby tagging along as a hopefully silent partner. Time your date to coincide with the baby's regular nap time, wheel the pram around until he nods off, and then enjoy an hour or so connecting with your partner over a nice meal. It can be so normalising and freeing to get out of the house sometimes.

Just don't have so much fun you forget to take the pram home with you when you leave. That would put a dampener on your date.

- **Day dates:** Babysitters can be *expensive!* If you return to work, and baby is in day care, you may consider having a day date. Leave work an hour or two early once a fortnight, before baby is due to be collected from day care. Meet your partner somewhere nearby day care and spend some quality time together before going in together to pick her up! Voila, free babysitting! (Especially if you can make the work hour up in lieu and don't have to take leave.)

- **Babysitters:** If you would like to head out on the town together, it can be tough, especially if you don't have family or friends around to babysit. Aside from the expense, it's super hard to consider leaving your baby home alone with someone you don't know well, or that your baby doesn't know well. Some day care educators babysit to make extra cash on the side. Because our son *loves* his day care teachers (as do we!) we feel completely comfortable leaving him with them for the night. He thought it was so cool to get his teacher all to himself while we attended a Christmas party!

Learn your partner's love languages

Relationship counsellor Gary Chapman struck relationship gold when he coined the idea of 'The 5 Love Languages'.[42] Basically, he advises that we must learn the way that our partner speaks and understands love, so that we can most effectively help them to feel loved. The five languages he describes are:

1. **Words of affirmation:** Praise, compliments, words of love and saying thanks are all examples of words of affirmation.
2. **Gifts:** Small, thoughtfully considered gifts, like bringing home a favourite flower, will mean a lot to the partner whose primary love language is gifts.
3. **Quality time:** Choosing to spend undistracted, quality time with your partner whose primary love language is quality time will help them to feel loved.
4. **Acts of service:** An example of actions speaking louder than words—the person with a primary love language of acts of service will feel loved when they come home to a cooked meal or a clean house.
5. **Physical touch:** The person who feels love through physical touch will appreciate physical gestures, like a back rub, or reaching for their hand as you drive in the car.

People often speak more than one love language, and it can be difficult when partners speak different languages. Often, one partner feels like they are expressing love *all the time* and it goes completely unnoticed, because their partner doesn't understand their spoken language. One partner may complain of feeling ignored and unloved because they haven't had much *quality time* from their partner, who is too busy trying to make them feel loved by *acts of service*—cooking dinner and cleaning the house! It's important to learn and understand each other's love languages.

Practise your communication skills

Try to be aware of the way you are communicating and the presence of any poor communication within your partnership. Consider writing in your journal when a fight blows up. Write down what you noticed. Were you happy with the way you were treated, and the way you treated your partner during this interaction? Did it feel respectful? Are there areas of communication either of you could improve on?

Make time to talk and then listen. Listen, listen and then listen some more. Listen with the sole intention of understanding. *Do not* plan what you are going to say next while you are listening—if you are doing that, you aren't really listening!

If there are problems within the relationship, address them as soon as possible. Try not to let things build up. Tackle things as they come up. As you saw in the couples' stories above, the partners had very different ideas about what was wrong in the relationship. Lots of things can be solved with open, honest communication.

Practical support

Consider splitting up the household jobs. Usually each partner has chores and tasks that they hate and chores that they don't mind. Consider splitting up regular chores, so that each partner is responsible for some of the everyday type tasks that need to get done. And then, of course, actually do them. But have grace towards each other, too. Sometimes life gets in the way, and things don't get done. That's okay. The problem occurs when one person picks up all the slack, all the time. That's not okay.

Reflection

Time to grab your journal again! Let's take a few minutes to think about your relationship with your partner, if you have one. You may even like to discuss this section with them, and it's completely up to you whether you do or don't.

- How is the communication between you and your partner? Has anything changed post-baby? Are there any communication issues that you can see were there before, but have become more noticeable since baby? Consider talking about these with your partner.
- What types of things would you like to do with your partner? What types of things will be possible to do at this very busy time of life? Are any of the above dating ideas possible for you?
- What can you do to lavish love on your partner this week? Remember to consider the types of things they like when coming up with ideas.
- What love language do you think you, and your partner, speak?
- What types of things would you like your partner to help more with at home? Or vice-versa? Have you considered splitting up chores and tasks according to what you each like doing?

11

On Postpartum Anger: What we don't talk about

When I became a mum, I also became, let's say, temperamental. It would take next to nothing to set me off. I was on edge and tense *all the time*. You know those people you walk on eggshells around, because anything you say or do can be taken the wrong way and used against you? That was me! I've always been slow to anger, but the postpartum period seemed to bring out my more Hulk-like tendencies. I have a new frown line on my face that I attribute to this time.

I hated it. I so didn't want to be that person. But I was.

Lots of the mums I spoke to told me that they, too, had felt extremely angry when their babies were small. In fact, it was one of the most common challenges they spoke about. In one way I was relieved to discover that this is a common experience postpartum. But while I was relieved that this was a thing, I was saddened to learn that so many of us suffer it silently. As has been stated often, the common challenges associated with new motherhood are not often spoken about, and this is especially apparent in this area. Why?

While there is still a stigma attached to mental health issues in general, being sad or anxious is becoming more normalised every day. People are working on reducing the stigma attached to being a sad mum or a scared mum. It's becoming more acceptable to be sad or scared. People understand and encourage women to seek the help they need. This is so great, so important, and yet . . . it's somehow not okay to be an angry mum. In our worst-case scenario brains, we envision that we could have our kids removed from our care. We feel like failures for getting angry with our kids. Because no one talks about it, we think that we are alone in our struggles, like no one else acts like we act.

Feeling anger towards our kids, especially when they are just babies, is something that new parents hide. But it is not an uncommon experience. And hiding it can stop people from getting the help they need. Hiding it means we fight it alone.

Feeling angry is normal. It's genetically wired into us. We spoke earlier about the fight or flight response; anger is part of that response—the fight part. When we are faced with a threat, whether it is a real or a perceived threat, a physical threat or an emotional threat, we respond. Some of us respond with our fight reflex. Our muscles tense, our heart rates increase, our breathing quickens, and we feel like fighting. It's a survival mechanism, a way of keeping our contribution to the human race alive.

Rage may be a more accurate description than anger of the way new mums can feel when they get overwhelmed. Rage is anger so intense that we don't feel in control of it. It's not like us, our 'normal selves', but we feel powerless to stop it.

I've spoken to several mums about anger and rage in their first year postpartum. Often, mums felt ashamed to talk about the issue. They thought they were the only ones who had felt the way they did and, more importantly, acted the way they did. I heard so many mums' stories about rage when their kids were babies. I've included some below, but there were *so many more*. These mums all had something in common: they were still feeling shame about it, weeks, months or even years later. Many of them had never spoken about these feelings with anyone before. All were relieved to hear that the feelings they were having were 'normal'.

Anger is an emotion, like any other emotion—sad, scared or happy. It's a bit different though. It's often referred to as a 'secondary emotion'. This is because people tend to get angry as an automatic response covering up another, more vulnerable emotion. The 'primary emotion' is the one you are experiencing *underneath* the anger. It's as though our brains are trying to protect us from our more vulnerable state. For me, anger often appears when I am feeling overwhelmed or anxious. I feel threatened and my body reacts—it gets ready to fight.

We know that feeling anger is normal, a normal secondary emotion, designed for survival. But our bodies haven't quite evolved to the point of being able to distinguish real, physical threats from emotional or perceived threats. Feeling angry isn't bad. Everyone feels angry sometimes. It's how we behave that matters—how we respond when we start to feel our primary emotions, whether anxiety, or sadness, or stress, when we feel ourselves getting angry. This is what matters to our babies, not that we were feeling angry in the first place. Babies aren't mind readers! They see what we do, not what we think. Anger is okay; aggression is not.

We need to identify what primary emotions are behind our anger. Do you tend to 'snap' when you are anxious, overwhelmed, sad or jealous? Any other primary emotions spring to mind? Perhaps you notice that you get angry when you experience a variety of any or all of these? Later we will work on identifying our primary emotions, our first anger signs and our triggers.

Why do we get angry?

Research has identified many things that contribute to postpartum anger and rage.[43] We can feel angry when our expectations don't match our realities. A mum who really wants to breastfeed and has trouble doing so, for example, and ends up feeding her baby formula. Her expectations of herself as a mother don't align with the reality she faces. A mum, who thought she would have lots of free time during her eighteen-week maternity leave and that she might even write a book during that time, had expectations about new motherhood that weren't ever going to align with the reality. (She shall remain unnamed—okay, yes, that was me!)

Mums also tend to feel angry when we feel powerless. Having a new baby at home does limit us, in ways we might not have been expecting. The simple things that up until yesterday we used to take for granted become 'mission impossible': going to the toilet, showering, sleeping enough, eating enough, exercising. We can feel trapped and powerless to the demands of new motherhood, especially while we are still adjusting. Rest assured, you will find your way, and soon this will be your new normal. You will gain back some semblance of control over your life. But it is normal to feel powerless at the beginning while you are adjusting, and this can contribute to feelings of anger in new mums.

Lack of support from others is also a big contributor to anger in new mums. We might perceive a lack of support from our friends or family members who we expected would be around more or do more to help us. We might feel that our partners aren't supporting us enough. We may even feel unsupported by medical staff.

Anger can also be caused simply by the lifestyle typical of a new mum: hormone fluctuations, lack of sleep and exhaustion, not eating well or enough—think lots of sugar and caffeine—lack of 'me time' and a lack of exercise. Do not underestimate the value of self-care.

What are the effects of anger?

Postpartum anger can occur on its own, or as a symptom of postpartum depression or anxiety.[44] Postpartum depression and anger are linked. Anger can prolong an episode of depression, and vice-versa.

Prolonged or intense anger can affect our relationship with our children. Sometimes mums are afraid of directing their anger towards their babies, so we put some distance between us and our kids, to protect them. This can affect how we bond with them, and even our long-term relationships with them.[45]

Our relationships with our partners can also be affected by chronic anger and rage. This is particularly evident if we don't talk to our partners about the way we're feeling.

Her story: Bree

Bree describes her pre-baby self as easy-going and carefree. A few weeks after giving birth, though, Bree said she felt like she had completely changed. She said she felt like a monster, always on the edge of completely 'raging out'. The smallest things would send her over the edge—the house being messy, dog hair on the couch, her baby crying. Bree felt like she was constantly either yelling or quietly seething, feeling the bubbles of repressed anger poisoning her from the inside out.

She knew sleep deprivation and hormones were contributing to this but didn't think there was a lot that could be done about it, so she continued to seethe. One day, she saw a friend who had had a baby at around the same time as her. Her friend was talking about going on a date night with her husband, and her baby was going to be left with her friend's parents who lived nearby. Bree didn't have any family nearby. She felt jealous, and she said she just suddenly felt like anger bubbles, which had been repressed for weeks, rose up and exploded out of her. She didn't know why, but she suddenly *hated* her friend. Bree suddenly thought her friend was the most annoying person on the planet, and she couldn't stand her.

She swore at her friend, telling her it must be nice to have her 'perfect life', and grabbed her baby more roughly than intended. She stormed off to her car and left her friend behind. Later she apologised, explaining that she didn't know where that came from, and her friend understood. But Bree still feels scared of the way her emotions overtook her that day, the way she hurt her friend and was rougher than intended with her baby.

Her story: Tamara

When Tamara's daughter was four months old, Tamara recalls a particularly bad night. The baby had had her vaccinations that day and was having an awful night. She was inconsolable, and Tamara could not settle her or get her to sleep. She had tried everything she knew. She said she was exhausted, overwhelmed and anxious that she would not be able to get her to stop crying at all, let alone get some sleep. Tamara remembers clenching her teeth and her fists, her heart racing, and rocking the baby harder and harder, patting her on the back with a bit more force than she usually did. It felt to her like the anger was rising in her chest.

While Tamara was aware that she was beginning to be forceful with her baby, she said it was like she couldn't control it. She did eventually set the baby down in her cot, not feeling safe about the way she was feeling, and went to wake her husband up to take over the settling. She knew that if she had stayed in that scenario, she was going to lose her temper.

Her story: Maria

Maria returned to her work as a physiotherapist when her baby was three months old. One morning before work, she was making breakfast for herself and her partner, and heating up a bottle at the same time. Her partner was holding the baby, who they had had to wake up so that they would all be ready in time for day care and work and the baby was screaming. Maria was getting more and more agitated and she had a headache. She started thinking about how unfair it was that she was already back at work, and silently blaming her husband for not earning more money so that she would be able to stay home longer. She felt 'stuck' in her circumstances and could feel the anger building.

Maria started to feel hot. The baby kept crying, and Maria saw that her husband had stopped trying to console the baby and was checking his phone! That was the last straw for her. She no longer felt she was in control of her actions. She opened the microwave, *slammed* the door shut, and threw the bottle at her husband—hard. Milk flew everywhere, and the bottle was way too close to hitting her baby's head. Maria couldn't believe that she reacted like that, and she feels a lot of guilt around that day.

Let's get practical

As we discussed in both our depression and our anxiety chapters, Chapters 8 and 9, when our fight or flight reflex has been activated (in this case, fight) it is impossible to switch off by force of will alone—remember me in the MRI machine in the anxiety chapter! Instead, there are behavioural strategies we must engage in to allow our logical brains to take over system control—and calm down our emotional brains.

One problem with anger intervention is that anger is an emotion with a very short lead time, in that it is quick to activate after a trigger. The adrenaline caused by activation of the fight or flight reflex is *fast* acting. This means that we need to be aware of our earliest anger signs in order to intervene as quickly as possible.

Common early anger signs include:

- jaw clenching
- teeth grinding
- feeling hot
- tummy troubles
- headaches
- sweating
- becoming shaky or dizzy
- fists clenching
- face turning red.

Next time you lose your temper, consider writing down in your journal what you can remember about the way your body felt immediately before that. Soon you will have a better idea of your early warning signs so that you can intervene as soon as possible.

Why am I angry?

It is necessary to identify things that are likely to trigger us—make us angry. This way we can be forewarned and forearmed before we even notice our early anger signs. Perhaps there is a way of avoiding some of our triggers before they become a problem; but not always—for example, you can't, for obvious reasons, avoid it if your baby crying is a trigger, but you might be able to if having a messy kitchen is a trigger.

Consider writing in your journal each time you notice yourself feeling angry or behaving in an aggressive way. Write down everything you can remember: what happened to set you off, what you thought, how you felt, what you did, what were the consequences of your actions? Write down your experience honestly—this is just for your eyes. It will help you to see the things in your life that may be contributing to your anger. It will also help you to objectively look at the way you are behaving when you do feel angry, and to see what the consequences of those behaviours were. Awareness is the first step to recovery, and this awareness will help you to make a better plan around responding to angry feelings.

Remove yourself from the situation

It sounds obvious, but just walking away is the most helpful thing you can do when you notice your early warning signs of anger. It is highly dependent on context, and most people find that their anger is somewhat alleviated by leaving the situation. Walk away and engage in some deep-breathing, grounding or mindfulness activities (see Chapter 9, 'On Postpartum Anxiety' for help with how to do these) in order to switch over system control of your brain to your logic centre. Or, if you find that too hard right now—perhaps you are too far down the anger path and the adrenaline is already surging—go for a brisk walk or do some star jumps. You need to basically work off some of the adrenaline that is present due to activation of the fight or flight reflex.

If you are angry with your baby—and this is common, so don't beat yourself up—and you begin to feel your early warning signs, it is much safer for you to leave your baby in a secure space, like their cot, and walk away for a five-minute breather to regain control, than to stay and try to 'push through it'. It is okay if your baby cries—you know they are safe, and you are doing the right thing. You will be back soon once you have calmed down.

The 'your turn' rule

If your partner or another support person is around when you begin to feel your anger signs, and you are finding it hard to control your temper, activate a 'your turn' rule. If you have spoken to your partner about your feelings, you can warn them that they need to respond when they hear the words 'your turn'. This way they will immediately understand what you are saying, without you needing to spell it out. 'Your turn' is code for, 'I'm feeling overwhelmed and you need to take over now!'

Let anger out (in the right way)

Repressing anger is *never* a good idea. But the methods that pop psychology tends to endorse about 'venting' our anger are *not* helpful either. Ideas such as punching and screaming into pillows, hitting a punching bag with the face of the person you are angry at pinned on it, and bopping each other with padded baseball bats abound in the mainstream media and in pop psychology— and indeed in real psychology practices in the past! But it turns out that behaving like an angry person makes us more likely, not less, to think and feel like one.[46] (Remember the cognitive behaviour therapy or CBT cycle in Chapter 8?) Research has shown that it is important to vent our anger but not in a violent, aggressive way. Physical activity, such as punching a boxing bag, is great, but not with a person's face on it! Baseball bats are great too, but hit a ball, not a person. A run is just as effective. Essentially, we don't want to strengthen our angry neural connections by watering the seeds of anger.

Progressive muscle relaxation

Progressive muscle relaxation (PMR) is another great way to release some anger and tension, calm our bodies down and re-engage our logical brains. PMR is a great way to reconnect with your body. It works by asking you to progressively work your way up your body, tensing and then relaxing all the different muscle groups. This helps you to become familiar with the feeling of being tense versus being relaxed, and to learn how to relax your body, which you will then begin to do automatically when your anger starts bubbling up.

To do this exercise, find a comfortable chair to sit in or lie down on your bed, a couch or the floor. Take a few slow, deep breaths—in through your nose, out through your mouth. Close your eyes if you prefer. The aim is to tense each muscle group for a period of five seconds, and then to relax the muscle group for a period of ten seconds.

- **Feet:** Point your toes towards the floor. Hold the tension for five seconds. Relax your feet. Point your toes up towards your head. Relax.
- **Hamstrings:** With bent knees if you are lying down, push your feet down into the ground. Hold. Relax.
- **Thighs:** Stretch your legs straight out in front of you and tense your thigh muscles. Relax.
- **Stomach:** Draw your belly button in towards your spine. Relax.
- **Back:** Arch your back. Relax.
- **Neck:** Bend your neck forward towards your chest. Relax.
- **Shoulders:** Draw your shoulders up to your ears. Relax.
- **Eyes:** Scrunch your eyes shut, closed tightly. Relax.
- **Forehead:** Wrinkle your forehead by opening your eyes wide and raising your eyebrows. Relax.
- **Upper arm:** Bring your hands to your shoulders and tense bicep muscles. Relax.
- **Wrists:** Bend your hand back. Relax.
- **Hands:** Clench your hands, the left one then right. Relax.

Also effective is talking about your feelings, or even writing a letter—though you are probably in no mood to do those last two things until your logical brain has regained control.

Once you have engaged in some physical activity and/or relaxation exercises to regain some control, or at a time when you feel calm, you will want to look at some of the thoughts (cognitions) that you are having. Angry thoughts lead to angry feelings, which lead to angry behaviours, so challenging some of our angry thoughts and beliefs is an important step in beating our aggressive behaviour long-term.

Common unhelpful angry thinking habits

We have discussed CBT and unhelpful thinking habits in the depression and anxiety chapters—please do go back and review these. CBT strategies are very helpful in coping with anger and rage as well, and most of the strategies in this section, indeed in this whole book, are CBT aligned. Some further examples of common unhelpful thinking habits that angry people may have are:

- **Personalisation:** An angry person tends to take things personally. They believe that people are out to get them or are judging or criticising them. They often have a 'victim' mentality.
- **Overgeneralisation:** When we overgeneralise, we are taking a few examples and imposing them across our whole lives and futures. When something goes wrong, for instance, an angry mum might think 'of course this happened to me; nothing ever goes right for me. I must be cursed'.
- **Mind reading:** Angry people are *frequent* mind readers, but often they are not that *good* at it. They usually infer

untrue negative thoughts on behalf of others. A mum whose partner has just gotten home and asks how her day was, might assume that he is asking because he has noticed that the dishes aren't done and dinner isn't on the table, and she then may begin to feel angry with her partner for his perceived 'thoughts'.

- **Black-and-white thinking:** Someone who is a black-and-white thinker may have trouble in their relationships because they see things as wrong or right, good or bad, and struggle with the in-betweens. They find it hard to communicate and to compromise on their own, usually rigid, beliefs. They feel angry when things don't align with their inflexible expectations.

- **Perfectionism:** Perfectionists tend to be quick to anger. They expect too much of both themselves and others. When their standards inevitably aren't met, because no one is perfect, they can feel badly let down, and this can turn into anger.

- **Emotional reasoning:** This is where we think because we *feel* a certain way it means something *is* a certain way. If we feel angry then it means that somebody has done something *really* bad to us. This justifies our anger to ourselves, and thus perpetuates it.

It is important to challenge these unhelpful thinking habits, and to strategically engage in more positive, rational and balanced thinking in order to form new neural connections. This will get easier over time. For now, it will take some strategic practice.

Consider challenging this anger by using the Thought template from Chapter 9. The example here will guide you—remember, no opinions or guesses are allowed during this activity. Facts only!

The Thought
Example: My partner is judging me for not getting dinner on the table or the dishes done; he has no idea how hard it is here at home with the baby; he's always like this

Evidence FOR the Thought	Evidence AGAINST the Thought
He asked how my day was I haven't done the dishes or made dinner	He asks me how my day was every day, even when I have made dinner and done dishes He didn't say anything about the dinner or dishes I also usually ask him how his day was He's not always like this; he rarely comments on things like dinner, and last night he made dinner

The Verdict
He is simply asking how my day was because he cares, and it's something he always asks. I am interpreting this as judgement because I'm feeling defensive; because I would have liked to get all my chores done and I am feeling like I'm failing at this mum stuff.

Dealing with anger is important

There is a story I like to tell my clients when they are struggling with anger. The author is not known, but it is a commonly referenced story about the lasting effects of anger.

There once was a little boy who had a bad temper. His father gave him a bag of nails and told him that, every time he lost his temper, he must hammer a nail into the back of the fence. The first day the boy banged 37 nails into the fence. Over the next few weeks, as he learned to control his anger, the number of nails hammered daily gradually dwindled down. He discovered it was easier to hold his temper than to drive those nails into the fence.

Finally, the day came when the boy didn't lose his temper at all. He told his father about it and the father suggested that the boy now pull out one nail for each day that he was able to hold his temper. The days passed, and the young boy was finally able to tell his father that all the nails were gone. The father took his son by the hand and led him to the fence.

He said, 'You've done well, my son, but look at the holes in the fence. The fence will never be the same. When you say things in anger, they leave a scar just like this one. You can put a knife in a man and draw it out. It won't matter how many times you say I'm sorry, the wound is still there, and a verbal wound is just as bad as a physical one.'

I've included this story here, not to say that if you've been angry then there is no redemption or that you will have forever scarred your loved ones, but to highlight the importance of seeking support or making changes if you find you are becoming angry a lot. I know there are things that I've done and said in anger that I wish I hadn't and that continues to play on my mind. As we discussed, this can lead to guilt, relationship issues, or trouble bonding with your kids. If you've discovered a reason you've been feeling angry—unmet expectations, lack of support, or feeling powerless perhaps—it is important to talk to your support network, to collaborate on ideas to help you out. If these things change, it is likely that your anger levels will improve too. If things continue the way they are, it's likely that some 'holes in the fence' may appear.

Manage your expectations

As one of the most common causes of anger is unmet expectations, we need to do some work on managing these expectations—both of ourselves and others. Things may not be the way we expect them to be, but the fact is, things *are* this way for now, and this is what life is for the moment. Some things we can change, perhaps by gathering support, or talking about our feelings, but some things are just the way it is for now—the nature of new parenthood. How are we going to make the very best of the life we have now, rather than dwelling on the past, or worrying about the future? Remember the Eckhart Tolle quote from page 43?

> Always say 'yes' to the present moment. What could be more futile, more insane, than to create inner resistance to what already is?

What could be more insane than to oppose life itself, which is now and always now? Surrender to what is. Say 'yes' to life—and see how life suddenly starts working for you rather than against you.

There is amazing value in learning contentment in our realities. Pushing back against what 'is' is a leading cause of anger and frustration—and it won't elicit any change in this case anyway!

Forgive—don't harbour resentment

One of my favourite sayings is by Malachy McCourt: 'Resentment is like taking poison and hoping the other person dies.' Another, by Lewis B. Smedes speaks the same message: 'To forgive is to set a prisoner free, only to discover that the prisoner was you.' Bad stuff might have happened to you. You might have every right to be angry. You also have every right to be free. Holding on to resentment and anger is only harming yourself, and you don't deserve it. For your sake, consider forgiveness.

This does not mean that you have to forget, or even see the person or people again to tell them that you forgive them. They don't even need to know—unless you think it would help you. You might write a letter you do or don't send, you might write a story that you then burn in a bonfire as a symbolic gesture of 'letting go', or you might simply choose to try to stop thinking about what happened, or the person who made it happen. You might use mindfulness strategies to help you with that goal. However you choose to 'let go' and forgive, I think that you will find it a freeing experience.

Reflection

Now it's your turn! Get your cuppa and your journal. Please try not to be ashamed, mama; this space is just for you, so please feel free to be completely transparent. If you do experience anger and rage, as you can see, you are not alone!

- What are your earliest anger signs?
- When you look at your journal, what do you notice are your common anger triggers? Did you notice patterns in what caused you to feel angry? What did you notice about the way you responded, and what the consequences of those responses were?
- Do you recognise any of these unhelpful thinking habits in yourself? They are pretty common! Consider doing the thought challenging exercise.
- If you have acted out in rage, how do you feel now? Have you spoken to anyone about this?
- How does it feel to know you are not alone and that being angry is a common symptom of postpartum?
- What would it look like to forgive yourself and move forward? Is there something stopping you?
- Is there anyone else that you would like to forgive and set yourself free from? How will you do that?

12

On Identity: Becoming Mum, staying me

I doubt that I'm the first person who has been propelled into an identity crisis by spending time on social media, and I doubt I'll be the last. It has a way of forcing self-examination and the creation of an online 'story' about one's self that can lead to feeling, well, let's call it 'less than'. Staring at the 'About Me' section of my Facebook page some three months after my son was born filled me with a sudden anxious introspection. Who even am I? How would I describe myself? I wrote 'Mum'—and then drew a mental blank.

Wait—that can't be all I am! A few months ago, I didn't even have any kids, so surely I must be more than Mum? I wasn't no one before having my son! I wrote 'Psychologist'.

But wait—if I had have chosen a different career path all those years ago, if my high school psychology teacher hadn't told me I had a 'knack for psychological jargon' (I still haven't figured out whether that was a compliment or not) and set me on this path, would I be a completely different person? Also, I was on maternity leave so I wasn't even currently 'psychologising'. (That's what my husband calls it—'Stop psychologising me!')

I had to be a person outside of what I did for work, and the fact that I had recently procreated.

What is a person's identity? Sure, it is made up of things such as what we do for work and our relationships—wife, mother, sister, friend. It also includes things such as our strengths, our values, our interests, our skills, our passions, what we contribute to others and the world. It includes our personality types, our temperaments and our health. It is a combination that is unique to us. At the risk of sounding like a greeting card, there is no one exactly like you!

No matter how much you doubt yourself some days, the fact is that you are completely individual, and you can do things that no one else in the world can do. Just think about that for a sec. You can do things that the most famous and talented people in the history of the world could not do—just because you are you.

Sometimes in life, let alone when we delve into the world of parenthood, we forget that. Sometimes we never knew it in the first place.

Let's focus on you—what you're good at, how you function best, what you enjoy, what you're passionate about, and what keeps you motivated. All too often when we become mums we do start to focus less on these things. We do this sometimes out of necessity—think time, responsibilities and complete and utter exhaustion—but I think also sometimes out of large-scale societal beliefs that when we become parents our needs matter less. Or don't matter at all. In becoming parents, we talk about 'losing' our identity. But that's impossible! We are still us, we exist and we matter. But sometimes we forget that we do.

One day when my son was two, I forgot to get ready for work—true story. I just forgot! I had made breakfast for my son—Vegemite on toast, we're not fancy—carefully packed his bag and ironed his clothes. I'd done the dishes, cleared the toys, paid a bill and fed the dog. Nearing the time that we were supposed to be out the door, my son said, 'You go work in your pyjamas, Mummy?' That's when I realised it: I'd forgotten to get ready for work. New low.

Talking to other mums I noticed something. I was not the only one whose needs were being lost in the chaos of life. This was a definite theme!

Some major themes of 'self-loss' ran through my conversations with mums, so I've split this chapter into sections: values, identity, temperament and self-care.

Values

What are your values? Yes, *your* values. Not your partner's, your children's or your mothers' group's. Yours! It's a pretty broad question, granted, but one that is so vitally important in our daily lives. Yet, it's a question that many of us spend little or no time at all thinking about. What we value should and could be a huge part of who we are but sadly often isn't, especially after we become parents. This concerns me.

When we live in a manner that is inconsistent with our values, or we spend too much of our time and mental energy thinking about things that we don't really value, we live in a state called 'cognitive dissonance'. Cognitive dissonance is a theory proposed by psychologist Leon Festinger.[47] It basically refers to that sense of mental unease or discomfort that occurs when our thoughts, beliefs and behaviours aren't aligned with each other.

As humans, we are constantly (consciously but often subconsciously too) seeking consistency across our thoughts, beliefs, opinions and behaviours. Take Sharon, a 46-year-old nurse, as an example of this. She strongly values health and wellness, yet she started smoking when she was a teenager, and is highly addicted. She smokes during her breaks at work and feels ashamed when her patients see her smoking outside the hospital. She feels like a hypocrite. She spends a lot of her workdays worrying that she might smell of cigarettes. In addition to worrying about what other people may think, she also can't understand why she keeps engaging in a behaviour that she knows is bad for her, even though she feels strongly about people living their best, healthiest lives—so much so that she has committed her life's work to it. Sharon is living in a state of cognitive dissonance.

Sharon has two choices if she wishes to achieve consistency across her thoughts, beliefs and behaviours. She can attempt to alter her thoughts and beliefs—perhaps she may try justifying them, as in if she were to quit smoking now, it is likely that she would put on weight, which has also been found to be a health hazard. Conversely, she can alter her behaviour to align more authentically with her beliefs, by quitting smoking. In this example, the latter option is quite clearly the better choice.

But as mums, new mums especially, we often get unwittingly thrust into a state of cognitive dissonance for reasons seemingly outside our control.

A mum who highly values her fitness and health, and engaged in a health-focused, active lifestyle pre-baby, may feel that state of cognitive dissonance, of mental unease, when she suddenly finds it hard to find time—and energy—to attend the gym and to prepare healthy meals for herself—or indeed meals at all. (Baked beans on toast three nights in a row, anyone?) She may not feel she has the option of changing her behaviours. Maybe the baby does not settle in the gym crèche, or she is not ready to leave her there, or she is healing from a caesarean section or an episiotomy. Perhaps finances are a limitation post-baby, when they weren't before. Perhaps she is tired all the time and lacking energy and motivation. So, she is forced to either change her beliefs and opinions about the importance of fitness and health on her life, or to live in a state of cognitive dissonance.

Another example is a mum who highly values a 'gentle' approach to parenting and to all her relationships. However, due to severe sleep deprivation, a lack of support, a colicky baby who will not stop crying whatever she tries, and a fuse that is shortening by the minute, she finds herself snapping at her partner the minute they walk in the door from work. When she lost all her patience she yelled at her baby. She has tried to alter her behaviours to align with her authentic self and her values but to no avail, due to the mental overload and physical strains placed on her by new parenthood. She also can't justify her actions to herself or feel okay about the way she has been behaving towards other people lately. So, she lives in a state of cognitive dissonance. She is mentally uncomfortable—all the time.

Do you recognise yourself in any of these examples? Are you feeling uncomfortable with any of your behaviours or your lifestyle since becoming a mum? Are there inconsistencies that make you uneasy?

How do we know when we are living in a manner that is consistent with our values?

Well, first we must think about what our values are. In the 'Let's Get Practical' section below, I've included a—non-exhaustive, of course—list of values. Have a look through and think about which values you hold most strongly. Hint: people say that you can often look in two places to find out what your own values are—your calendar and your bank statement. As in, how you spend your time and how you spend your money.

Another way to determine whether we are living according to our values is to do a check of our own peace of mind and feelings. You know when you get that sense of peace, that everything is right in the world, and you just feel a genuine joy? Think about what you are doing in those moments. Perhaps chatting with a loved one, doing something kind and selfless for someone else, spending time in nature, tackling a task that is important to you. I bet you find that your activities in those moments reflect your own values. This is an example of you living a meaningful life, by bringing your core values into your everyday life. It doesn't take much extra effort to live a values-led existence—in fact it takes much less mental energy than trying to live an existence according to other people's values! But it can make all the difference to how you live your life and how you feel within it.

Remember, our values don't all look the same. There is no one-size-fits-all set of values and trying to focus on other people's values may make you miserable. Think about your own.

Living a values-led life does not mean that life will always be rosy. It doesn't mean you will be happy for all time and never have any problems. (I wish it were that easy!) What it does mean is that you will be living a meaningful life, the way you want to live, and dealing with things in a way that is right for you, even when things are difficult in your world. You are being true to yourself.

We often don't have a lot of time to devote to ourselves in new motherhood. This means we need to work out ways to bring our core values into our everyday lives. It needn't take a complete life overhaul to live a values-led life. A bit of awareness and some small tweaks can make a huge difference.

Identity

I mentioned before that I had faced a small, social media inspired identity crisis while trying to fill in my Facebook profile shortly after I had my son. I truly could not think of anything to write about myself, other than what I did for work and the fact that

I was a mum. Sure, some of that was sleep deprivation and baby-brain—gosh, I was *tired* back then! But it was also evidence of just how little I had been focusing on myself outside of mother-hood, for probably the last year, since I had become pregnant. I had forgotten that writing and storytelling were such a strong part of my soul, for instance. I used to lose whole days while I lay on my bed and scribbled until my hand cramped up and my eyes were glassy, and I used to wake up in the middle of the night, unable to get to sleep until I had gotten that story onto paper. When I had that realisation, staring at the computer screen, I made the decision to focus on a part of me that had been forgotten—writing. I immediately set up an entirely separate Facebook page, a writer's page, and began blogging. That was the day I felt myself start to return. I could be mum and still be me. I called my first blog 'She Writes to Exhale'—because I did! Writing is a part of my identity.

So, what is an identity? We discussed before that our identities are made up of many things: our careers and our rela-tionships, our strengths that come naturally and the skills we have acquired, our interests and passions, our personalities and temperaments. Like a fingerprint, no one has the exact replica of our personal identity. We are all one of a kind.

Let's focus a minute on our strengths, because often strengths are defined as simply things that we are good at. But they are more than what we are good at. We can be good at something that is *not* a strength. Sarah, as an example, is talented with numbers and became a successful accountant. But, while working as an accountant, she was ending each day feeling drained, unfulfilled and out of energy. She did not feel she was living a strengths-based life; rather, she felt that she had fallen into this work because she happened to be good with numbers in school. She felt stuck in a job that wasn't her. She did not see accountancy as her strength. However, she came to realise that she did enjoy working with people every day and that *that* was her strength—engaging with people and helping them in their everyday lives. She then chose to pursue a career that would allow her to do this in a way that was more aligned with her strengths—what she was good at but also what fuelled and energised her. She went on to study social work, and she feels very passionate about her work now.

Temperament—introversion/extroversion

Let's also speak about temperament; specifically, where we are on the introversion/extroversion spectrum. Our temperament can have a huge impact on our overall adjustment to parenthood, so it is important to consider.

An introvert is someone who gains their energy from inside themselves, whereas an extrovert gains energy from being around other people. As such, an introvert needs time to themselves to recalibrate and re-energise in between interacting with the world. The problem is, babies aren't great at 'me time'—it's always 'us time' with them! They are little social butterflies who are not great with boundaries and who have limited—okay, no—capacity to read social cues. They are fully reliant on us, as they are supposed to be. But it can be hard to reconcile an introverted temperament with the way we feel we 'should be' as a mum, and societal expectations of what being a good, involved mum looks like.

As I mentioned earlier, when my newborn son was napping my husband used to ask me if he could wake him up to play. He said he missed him. *Missed* him! I didn't even know how to respond. Why didn't I miss my son while he was napping? Why was I so thrilled to finally get some alone time that I'd practically skip out of the room when I'd managed the miraculous car to cot transfer? Why, when I was looking forward to some solo time while my hubby took bub shopping, and he asked me if I wanted to come with them to the shops, would I not even need to think about it for a second before responding, 'No thanks'. Was I a horrible, selfish, cold-hearted shell of a person, who didn't love her son? Not at all! I couldn't have been more in love with him. But I am an introvert who desperately needs time alone to recharge my proverbial batteries. With a newborn, this time is so hard to come by. You relish it when you can.

On the other hand, a strongly extroverted person may also struggle with the adjustment to parenthood. Spending lots of time at home with a new baby, perhaps being home from work, with less time to engage in hobbies and having less social interaction overall, may lead to a feeling of isolation and a lack of energy for the extroverted parent.

Whatever way you are wired, it is possible to parent and live in a way that is consistent with your temperament.

Self-care

If I had a dollar for every time someone told me to 'practise self-care' I'd have—well, probably only about $20, which isn't even enough to buy one of those sensory deprivation 'float' thingies. (How cool do they sound, though?) The point is, people said it a lot. How do we work self-care into our lives without having to make room for one more task on the to-do list? Health, fitness, relaxation—even 'me time' started to feel more like a chore to me than a break during new parenthood. Had these well-meaning people forgotten what it is like to have a new baby?

People often remark to new mums that 'the housework can wait' and tell them to focus on nothing but themselves and their baby. But the thing is, the housework can't wait, not really. Or rather, it has already waited—and waited and waited until there aren't any clean clothes to wear or dishes to eat off! At some point, it can't wait anymore—a sad reality. We need clean dishes to eat off, we need to clean our clothes and bed sheets—babies leak a *lot*, from every orifice—and we need food to eat. The bins need to go out and the bathroom needs to be hygienic. The floor needs to be clean enough to eat off, because your baby *will* eat off it. Some people feel uncomfortable and unable to relax if there is too big a mess in the house, and there's always *some* mess with a baby. For these people, advice to leave the mess until later makes them feel really anxious, like, 'Now I'm not only worrying about my messy house, but I'm also worrying that my priorities are bad and I'm not savouring my kid enough'. It's fine if part of your self-care routine includes housework, either doing it yourself or enlisting help. There is no right way to care for yourself. You've known yourself for long enough to know what does and doesn't work for you. But when do we do all the things?

Though we love our babies and are willing to make any number of sacrifices for them, it is crucial that we don't forego all our needs in the process of becoming a parent. Our happiness matters—and not just our happiness. Our overall mental health matters, too.

Here's where I ask you to recall the old self-care metaphor that we spoke about in Chapter 2. On an aeroplane, the flight attendants tell us to fit our own oxygen masks before attending to the needs of others, including babies and children. Why is this advised? Well, because you are no good to anyone if you stop breathing. But if it came to the crunch, how would it feel to actually follow the advice, watching your baby struggle to breathe, scared and wide-eyed and screaming for mummy, then spending precious seconds affixing an oxygen mask to your *own* face? Confronting, right?

It is confronting, but it is necessary, and it is for the ultimate good of your baby.

New parenthood and infancy are about developing a new, two-way relationship with another person. How much time did it take to really know your partner? Did you spend time letting them in on your needs, wants, passions, desires, values and quirks? Did you take the time to learn theirs? What would it have been like if you focused only on their needs and didn't try to communicate with them what you needed to live your best, most fulfilled life?

A respectful, two-way, authentic relationship between a parent and an infant requires our children to get to know us—the real us, not just the mum part of us. We start as we mean to go on. As we continue to prioritise our own self-care in the chaos of parent life, as we show our kids our real lives, our passions, our strengths, our friendships, and our wins, we give them permission to find their own. This is a positive step towards developing a mutual respect and an authentic relationship with each other.

I'm talking here about recognising and asserting our own place in our relationship with our infant. I'm talking about prioritising our own needs, even while we spend our days tending to our kids' needs. That may look like taking along our bundle of joy to the gym crèche—even if it is not their favourite pastime—so we can have that hour that we so desperately need to feel like ourselves again. It may look like our babies playing with some toys in their playpen while we take fifteen minutes to drink our cup of tea while it is still hot. It may look like spending that extra twenty minutes in the kitchen preparing a nutritious lunch for ourselves, rather than scoffing down a piece of bread while spending an hour pureeing antioxidant-laden veggies for our babies. It may look like leaving our baby with our partner, a grandparent or a babysitter while we attend our weekly netball game, choir meeting or art class—or, as I do, spending one a night a week just sitting in my 'writing room' with my husband taking care of our son. It might look like bringing our baby along for a lunch catch-up with a friend.

Self-care is not selfish, and it is necessary, to live our best lives.

But self-care isn't always about taking extra time to do whatever we need or want to do. It doesn't necessarily mean bubble baths, gym sessions and massages. Self-care should be interlaced throughout our ordinary daily lives. Making decisions about what we choose to put in our bodies, who we choose to spend our time with, what we choose to commit to, what we feed our minds with, these daily decisions are all a part of self-care. These seemingly simple decisions shape our everyday lives and the way we cope and function overall. We need to consider ourselves as well as our baby and family in our everyday decisions.

Absence of a village

We were never meant to do this whole parenting thing alone. There is a common saying, 'It takes a village to raise a child'. Indeed, in the past, until quite recently, the village was alive and well. Grandparents, aunties, cousins, neighbours—everyone pitched in to raise the village children. New mums would be cared for and tended to for months postpartum; they even got to sleep from time to time! Parents used to share life's pressures with an entire community of other parents and support people. They would tackle life's burdens and pressures as a team, sharing advice, childcare, chores, and basically doing life together.

This still happens in some parts of the world. In our modern Western society though, there are no villages. Or they are very limited. We get home each night, and drive into our individual driveways, our garage doors roll closed behind us, and we enter the four walls of the house. We probably haven't even laid eyes on our neighbours today. Extended families are much more likely to live far away from each other, or to have commitments, work and busy lives outside of the family.

This means that the mental, emotional and physical burden of parenting lies squarely on our shoulders alone. And it can be heavy. And isolating. We put so much pressure on ourselves to be an entire village to our children, to supply what an entire village used to provide—interaction, new experiences, learning opportunities, a sense of belonging, physical care, many and varied social connections. Self-care. Prioritising our relationship. The list is endless. We have no room left to be ourselves, to be true to our *own* identity. We are too busy being everything to everyone—doctor, driver, maid, confidant, friend, entertainment committee, chef, teacher. Where are we in all of this? Who even has time to think about that?

In addition, we crave social interactions, and the closest and most effective way of getting this as a new parent is often social media. This doesn't always end well and can lead us to feeling even more disconnected and inadequate. We compare ourselves and consider all we are *not* doing. Our self-esteem plummets but it is important to remember: you are not the problem. You are doing the best you can. The expectations we have on ourselves—and that society seems to have on us—are not realistic. We cannot do it all by ourselves. We were never meant to. We need a village.

Her story: Jodie

Jodie is a 27-year-old teacher and a first-time mum. When she first went on maternity leave, she struggled to say goodbye to her students and colleagues, knowing that she wouldn't be teaching for at least a year. Teaching was a huge part of Jodie's identity—she even played 'school-teacher' back in primary school, and constantly found herself helping her friends with their schoolwork in high school and university. It was who she was. She really valued knowledge and had a real strength for relaying knowledge to others patiently, and in easy-to-understand ways. She was also very creative and enjoyed spending time thinking up inspiring ways to get people interested in learning.

On maternity leave Jodie felt stifled under the monotony of everyday life. She missed having interactions with others, she missed being creative, and she missed teaching. She loved her baby, but she didn't feel like she was using her gifts or strengths in a meaningful way. She looked forward to her baby growing older and more interactive, but right now she felt drained and heavy at the end of each day. She didn't have much energy, so she spent most of her days in the house—she watched a lot of Netflix.

Jodie came to realise that what she was missing was the ability to live a life that fit her identity. She wasn't being creative, interacting with others, or using her strengths. Further, she came to realise that she could be, and that she wasn't restricted from doing that—it would just need to look a little different than before! She began to create little songs to sing to her baby at bedtime, and activities to do with her baby at 'tummy time'. She began organising for friends to come over for visits and taking baby to a local playgroup. She registered for some online personal development courses to do in her own time at her own pace.

Jodie found that these small changes, which allowed her to nurture parts of her own identity such as her extroverted temperament, her strengths and her values, really made a difference in her energy levels and her mood.

Her story: Mallory

Mallory finds herself completely overwhelmed. Her baby is three months old, and she feels like she hasn't had an hour to herself in all that time. When her baby goes to sleep at night, she can barely keep her eyes open and she falls into bed, exhausted, only to wake up a few hours later to feed the baby. When her baby naps during the day—he tends to 'catnap' and has several short sleeps a day—she rushes around trying to get the house clean and the washing done but never accomplishes all she set out to do, and so never sits down to relax.

She is fatigued, and says she has no energy left to even think about self-care. Mallory describes herself as 'touched out'—she can barely force herself to give her husband a kiss when he walks in the door from work, and anything more than that, forget about it. She describes herself as an introvert. She has always enjoyed solitary activities like reading, journaling and watching movies. When Mallory spends a lot of time surrounded by people, she comes to a point where she needs a break to recharge by herself.

She first noticed this about herself on school camps as a child, and it has continued throughout her life. Before having her baby, Mallory worked in an open-plan office and by Friday afternoon she was 'peopled out', looking forward to her Friday nights alone.

But she didn't expect to feel that way with her baby. She hadn't considered that she was about to spend every waking moment in the company of another human who is completely dependent on her. She hadn't considered her introverted temperament as a potential extra challenge. It is more draining than she would have expected.

Mallory spoke to her husband about this, after a particularly bad night when she had told him to 'get out of my space'. As a fellow introvert, and someone who had known Mallory for a long time, he completely understood, and when she explained her feelings he told her that 'everything clicked into place and made sense'.

She and her husband worked together to organise their days so that Mallory had some daily alone time, and a longer stretch of time on the weekends. She found that once this strategy had been implemented, she was more patient, and more able to be present in the moment with her husband and with her baby.

Let's get practical

A word on values

To live a meaningful life filled with purpose, we need to find ways to bring our core values into our everyday lives. Firstly, we need to consider what our values are. We do this by reflecting on times when we felt at peace, content and energised. When was the last time you felt this way? What were you doing? I bet that you were doing something that aligned with your personal values.

You may have been being creative, helping someone, focusing on your health, or doing just about anything. Your values are personal to you.

Your bank statement and your calendar are a good place to start looking to determine your values. Where do you spend your time, and on what do you spend your money? These things are likely to reflect your values. If they don't, then it's likely that you may be living in the uncomfortable state of cognitive dissonance, as we discussed before. Here is a list of examples of values:

- authenticity
- balance
- challenge
- citizenship
- community
- compassion
- contribution
- creativity
- equality
- fairness
- growth
- health
- learning
- popularity
- recognition
- religion
- respect

- social justice
- success.

This list is not exhaustive—you may think of others—but it will allow you to reflect on values and get you started in thinking about your own core values. Write them down in your journal.

Discovering our strengths

As well as our values, our identity encompasses our strengths. Our strengths are not solely what we happen to be good at, but also what interests us and energises us. This is a true strength. When we discover what our true strengths are, we can decide to use our strengths in our everyday lives, in a similar way that we have determined to live according to our values.

Think about what you are good at, what interests you, and what you feel passionate about. When was the last time you used that strength? Have you been living your best, strengths-based life, or have you been trying to fit yourself into a mould that just wasn't you? Rather than focusing on weaknesses and what you don't do well, or aren't interested in learning, consider how you can use your own personal strengths to accomplish the things you need and want to accomplish—both in parenthood and outside of it.

Stop comparing yourself!

A meaningful, purposeful, strengths-based life does not look the same for every mum, and you need to find your fit. Your own values, strengths, temperament and overall identity are personal to you, and this means that you will be worse at some things than other mums. And you will be better at some things than other mums. It's not a competition, but it can begin to feel like one when we are constantly comparing ourselves with others. We will always fall short in some areas, and unfortunately it is human nature to focus on the negatives rather than the positives—it's a survival mechanism. It takes a deliberate effort to focus on the good things but with practice it gets easier. Remember the watering seeds example from earlier in the book—seeds that are watered, have attention paid to them, are the ones that grow. Don't water negative comparisons.

Your temperament and you

Consider your temperament. Would you describe yourself as an introvert or an extrovert? Or perhaps somewhere in the middle? How do you feel when you have been around people for a long time? How do you feel when you have been by yourself for a long time? Drained, energised, peaceful, agitated? You may need to consider some strategies to implement to allow you to parent according to your temperament.

For introverts this may mean including some alone time into your week, with the help of a support network and/or partner. If this is not possible, you can get creative with ways to be alone. I used to take a walk with the pram every afternoon. Baby would be content looking at the world around him, sometimes he'd fall asleep, and I would either wear headphones and listen to music or a podcast, or just be alone with my thoughts. If you are an extrovert, you may like to integrate some more social interaction time into your weekly schedule where possible, even if that time is just a phone call.

Create a village

Stop pressuring yourself to be an entire village. You are just one person, and no one can do it all. The pressure to try to do this is driving us collectively crazy! Instead, ask for help. Reach out. Be vulnerable with people you trust. You will probably find that the people you choose to confide in are feeling a similar way to you. In the absence of a village in today's Western society, we tend to be struggling with loneliness, disconnection, fatigue and pressure. Then we compare ourselves, often via social media, and imagine that everyone has it together except us. A bit of transparency, vulnerability and openness with each other will help us to create villages of our own. The villages may not look they did in the past, but they will lead to connection, support, and take some of the load off—and isn't that the whole point?

Self-care

Practise self-care. And remember that self-care doesn't have to be one more thing added to the to-do list. Self-care won't help if it's a chore. It's not all about bubble baths and massages—definitely nothing against those things, though! Self-care should be intertwined throughout our everyday life in the decisions we make for ourselves. The things we put in our body, the things we choose to focus on, the people we choose to spend our time with, the activities we do—and don't—partake of. Self-care can look like assertiveness, saying no, saying yes, healthy eating and exercise, letting go of comparisons and negative thoughts, or making plans to suit your strengths and your temperament. It is the everyday decisions and practices that you engage in that make up your overall life, and the way you feel within it. If you consistently consider your own needs in making the everyday decisions, then you are caring for yourself in the best possible way.

Remember 'you' as well as 'mum'

Remember, you are an entire, complete person outside of being 'mum'. Consider yourself a year ago. What were you interested in and passionate about? What did you spend time doing? What did you contribute to the world around you? What were your goals? What did you see as your purpose? These things did not cease to exist when you became a parent, and they still matter! Though you may be focusing on treading water in this new parent phase, remember that you can be a mum and still be you. It's important that your baby sees the real you as she grows up—seeing you prioritise your values, strengths, needs, passions and relationships sets an example and gives her permission to do the same as she grows. It also helps you to be a much more content, energised and peaceful parent!

Reflection

- After reflecting on the strategies above, what do you see as your core values? What are some ways that you can incorporate these into your everyday life?

- Have you noticed any cognitive dissonance, any mental unease—do you think there is a discrepancy between your core values and your current way of life or behaviours? Why is that?

- What are your strengths? Things you are good at, but also interested in and passionate about? Do you get to use these much in life now? How could you begin to use them more, to live a strengths-based life, during this new-parent stage?

- What are some ways that you could care for yourself in a consistent, nurturing way, within the everyday decisions that you make?

13

On Work: Returning
to work (or not)

To return to work, or not to return to work: that is the question. Well, one of a plethora of questions often asked of new mums in their first year of motherhood. It is one of the major questions, nonetheless. When our paid maternity leave nears its end, we need to make the decision: Will I return to my paid job, seek paid work, or stay at home with my kid/s?

Parental leave

In Australia, we may be entitled to up to eighteen weeks of paid parental leave from the government, provided we meet some eligibility requirements. This consists of minimum wage payments from Centrelink of $719.35 per week, before tax (current information in March 2019). There is also 'dad and partner pay', which is two weeks of pay at the same rate. Parental leave is only paid while we are on leave. If we return to work early, we stop getting paid from Centrelink. Have a look at the Centrelink website or give them a call to check your eligibility. (Be prepared for a long wait if you do call—have a cuppa and a book handy. My record is 1.5 hours on hold. Man, I was busting for the toilet.)

Some workplaces offer additional paid parental leave as part of your employment package, so to find out what you are entitled to, have a look at your employment contract or talk to your work's personnel section. Employers are obligated to hold our positions, or at least a position on our level and at our pay rate, for a period of one year, and it is up to the individual employer whether any of that twelve months is paid or unpaid leave.

Within the government's paid parental leave scheme, we are entitled to up to ten 'keeping in touch' days. This can be a good opportunity to, as the name indicates, keep in touch with our workplace. We may use these days to attend conferences, meetings or professional development activities, or just do our normal work activities here and there so we don't forget how to, say, use the scanner, like I did! (In my defence, it is an unnecessarily complicated scanner.)

When you return to work after parental leave, if you choose to do so, it is legislated that employers 'consider' flexible working arrangements. This means that you are entitled to request a change in how you work, but not that your employer is mandated to approve your request. You may request the ability to work from home or to condense your full-time job into a four-day working week, and these arrangements may or may not suit your workplace and your job. Your employer is obligated to consider your ideas though, and if your specific ideas won't suit, they may offer other solutions.

The best thing to do is to make time for a good conversation with your employer so you can come up with a plan together. Flexible work arrangements are possible if both parties are amenable. Some jobs and workplaces are more suited to these than others. My job as a psychologist, for instance, would be very difficult to do from home, and so while these types of arrangements wouldn't be possible for me my work goes out of its way to provide flexibility in other ways.

To work or not to work

The number of mums who eventually return to work has steadily increased over the last decade, and in 2017 the Australian Bureau of Statistics reported that 64 per cent of couple families consisted of both parents working. Most commonly, one parent worked full time and one parent worked part time.[48]

This may be due to necessity—it can be difficult (understatement much?) to live on one income these days. Or it may be a choice, and more options are now available for flexible working arrangements, which is a positive step in the right direction for those who do work. But what is right for you?

For many mums—myself included—returning to work wasn't a choice, and it always feels like a bit of a kick in the teeth to hear about my 'choice' to be a working mum. In our own family's personal and financial situation, that was just the way it was always going to be, and so no decision had to be made. I don't mean to make it sound like every mum has the choice to stay at home in today's economic climate. They just don't. In fact, according to the ABS, many mums of small children work in paid jobs outside of the home, whether that be full time or part time.[49]

Shortly after I returned to work after my maternity leave, I attended a seminar on child development for my job. I was looking forward to it on both a professional and a personal development level, as well as for the buffet lunch. (Okay, mostly for the lunch!) But then the speaker started talking about potential risk factors for childhood development, and it was like he was listing everything I'd done as a parent. He spoke about formula feeding, about young babies attending day care while parents worked, about babies being premature, and about babies living far away from their extended families and grandparents. I felt like everyone in the room who knew me was looking at me! They weren't, of course—they were probably all thinking about all the ways they had stuffed up their own kids. (I joke, I joke!) I did feel like the worst mum ever for a minute there. As the man kept speaking he said it was okay, because for every 'risk factor' our babies face, we just need to implement a 'protective factor' and then we will 'break even'.

The protective factors he suggested were things like speaking several languages at home or learning a musical instrument. (Right, I'll just get right on that!) These things are wonderful, of course, but unfortunately, they weren't in my skill set, so I had no hope of teaching them to my six month old. After that day

I did, though, begin to research the risks and benefits for children based on whether parents work or stay home. That research is so conflicted—it's not black and white.

Lots of research studies find there is no difference in childhood development whether a parent stays home or goes to work. Lots of others also say that kids benefit from having stay-at-home parents. And lots more say that kids benefit from their parents working. I think the very last thing that we, as new parents, need to do is to wade through pages and pages of conflicting and contradictory ideas and 'evidence', especially when going to work or staying at home may not even be a choice you get to make in the first place, like me. Just know that either way, if your baby is loved, safe, and their needs are taken care of, everything will be okay.

I often give myself permission to wander off into imagination land and wonder whether, if I did have the choice, would I have been a working mum or a stay at home mum. (I try not to wander too far into that land, in case my imagination comes up with an answer I can't have—read: I want to stay at home and still have a million dollars of spare change in my back pocket.) The answer I come up with is this: I don't think I'm a good candidate for staying home full time.

I think some women are, they thrive, and they love it. But every woman is different, and those women aren't me. I might have chosen to return to work a bit later than I did with my son— when he was five months—or do less days per week—currently I do four—but I still would have returned. I love my job, I love the balance it provides me between home and work, I love that a huge part of my identity and what I am valued for is outside of the home, and I love the social aspect. I also love peeing in peace and drinking a cup of tea *while it is still hot*. It's lovely.

If you have the choice, you may be at the point of thinking seriously about what you're going to do next. Here are some points to consider around the issue.

- **Finances:** Ask yourself whether you can realistically afford to stay at home—or go to work. Would your lifestyle be compromised by not working and, if so, to what degree and what are you willing to sacrifice to stay at home with your kids? For some of us, any amount of financial sacrifice may be worth it, while others may feel uncomfortable and limited by the financial burden placed on them by becoming a stay-at-home mum. Conversely, with the cost of day care, some mums say that outweighs any income they would earn, so they can't afford to go to work. Everyone's situation is different.

- **What you want to do:** This is a point that women often ignore: what do *you* want to do? The only people who get a say in this decision are the people who are going to be affected by it—as in you and your partner, if you have one, and your child. (Obviously, they probably don't have much of an opinion at this point in their young lives!) Do you think you would go stir crazy being at home with your baby all day? Would you be risking career progression, the chance to express your talents and creativity, or your social life by staying home? Do you feel strongly and passionately about being able to stay at home with your baby? These are examples of questions to ask yourself when trying to determine what *you* want to do.

- **The benefits for you of paid work:** We've discussed the benefits for our baby of us going to work outside the home (or not). We also need to consider what benefits (if any) *we* experience by going to our paid jobs. Do you achieve mental, social, emotional stimulation? Would you miss that if you were to give up your paid job to be a stay-at-home mum, or would you still experience these things via working inside the home?

- **The future:** Even if we could afford it in the short-term, there may be long-term financial consequences to not working outside the home. Career progression, long-service leave, superannuation, losing skills and having to re-qualify. These are things to consider long-term when making the decision to continue to work in a paid job or to stay at home.

Challenges for the working mum

Time pressure

Sociologist Judy Rose completed an Australian study in 2017 in which she spent time conducting in-depth interviews with several working mums.[50] The overwhelming theme throughout her research was that working mums are one of the most time-pressured groups out there. We often tend to try different strategies to make life work for us, and run smoothly, such as multitasking, organisation, and flexible work arrangements. But it seems that these strategies only go a little way to help with our perceptions of time; specifically, there is never enough of it.

Working mums tend to do a lot at once. We might spend our lunch breaks at work paying bills, or talking to our kids' teachers on the phone, and we may multitask cooking dinner and answering work calls or emails. Today at work I simultaneously ate lunch at my desk, was on the phone on hold to my son's doctor and typed a report. We don't often tend to be at home without our children, so the housework is done in conjunction with childcare, and I can attest to the fact that vacuuming is a whole lot less efficient when I have to 'take turns' with my toddler, who has the worst case of FOMO I've ever seen. (But, I think, what a great opportunity to teach turn taking and sharing!) Every moment in life is accounted for, and filled to its maximum capacity. If we could find a way to fit more into our time, you can bet your bottom dollar we would try. We are drowning in our attempts at efficiency. No wonder we are exhausted.

Another interesting finding in Rose's research was that working mums' perceptions of time are 'warped'. During the days, especially in intense periods of multitasking and time pressure, time seems to stand still or speed up for us—usually in the opposite way to what we would prefer, of course! Working mums were also likely to look at spaces of time negatively. Seeing a block of time as 'empty' or 'inefficient', for instance. When time is so limited, we feel an immense pressure for each second to be well spent, and inefficiency or empty time can feel like a real waste. I can certainly relate to this! When every second of the day needs to be planned, organised and used wisely, lest it be seen by us as 'wasted', it can leave less room for us to live in the moment, practise self-care, or just enjoy life with our kids!

Mum guilt and worker guilt

Sometimes I feel like I am in a tug of war between home and work. This was particularly bad when my son was a baby. It was incredibly hard to hand my five-month-old son over to his carers in the morning. He looked so vulnerable, not even able to sit up on his own yet. I wondered if his carers knew him better than I did. I wondered if he would like them better than me or have more fun at day care than at home with me. I wondered if they did a better job than I did—after all, they were much more experienced with babies than I was. I wondered if some of the snarky comments I'd received were correct: were his day-care teachers actually raising him? (For the record, the answer to that is a firm no—you are a full-time mum who is raising your own child, regardless of whether you work or not.)

Then, I'd also feel guilty for missing meetings, or going home early when my son was sick. (By the way, this happens *a lot*, during their first year or so at day care—be warned.) I spent a lot of time 'in the red' on carer's and annual leave over the first two years of my son's life. I got a sinking feeling in my stomach when I had to tell my boss last minute that I wouldn't be in again. I felt like I wasn't concentrating or 'on my game' as much as previously, due to sleep deprivation and the general juggle of competing demands that come along with mum life. No matter whether I was at work or at home, I felt like there was somewhere else I should be.

Challenges for the stay-at-home mum

24/7 work hours

As a stay-at-home mum, the hours are relentless. You're on 24/7 with no pay, no set lunch breaks, or even solo toilet breaks! Your days are determined by your baby, and your breaks may be contingent on what mood he is in today. He can be a demanding boss! Parenting is a full-time gig no matter whether you go outside the home to work or not but stay-at-home mums are doing the *same* job all day and all night. There may be (but not always) less shared responsibility in the home, with housework, life administration, and so on. Because mum is at home it's all seen as 'her job'. Of course, dads can stay home too, and face these same issues, but mums do tend to take on this role more often. It's important that partners (if there is a partner) work together to ensure that stay-at-home parents get a break from their job. I cannot stress this enough. Many mums who stay home reported that the best gift they could be given is just an hour a day to themselves. One hour! Many said it would be life changing. This is do-able, isn't it, partners?

Disconnection

Some stay-at-home mums have commented to me that they feel a sense of loneliness or disconnection by staying home. Though most women are happy with the decision they've made to stay home, they are finding themselves lonely and somewhat isolated, particularly if most of their social connections do go out to work during the day. As would be expected, mums who have a support network of other mums who stay home don't tend to feel this way as much.

Tangible achievement

Some mums commented that they felt like they had never been busier in their lives than when they were staying at home with their baby, but that they never felt as though they had achieved anything. They may have cooked, cleaned, run errands, changed nappies, provided entertainment and fed their baby all day, but at the end it was as though nothing was achieved. By this, I mean, it all needed to be done again tomorrow. In fact, they had achieved a lot—they had nurtured, cared for, loved and developed their baby! But because their work was never 'done' they spoke about not feeling a sense of 'accomplishment' at the end of the day. Some mums missed that about working outside the home, and it had started to wear on their sense of self. *Especially* when they heard the most aggravating question in the world for the hundredth time: 'So what do you *do* all day?'

Her story: Karen

Karen is a single mum. She returned to work after her eighteen-week government maternity leave—her work didn't provide any extra leave. She didn't feel quite ready to return to work, but financially it was the only option for her. She had a good job that she liked, and although she wasn't sure she was ready, she was looking forward to some aspects of working again—she had missed her colleagues over the last few months.

Her first day back at work was hard. She dropped her son off at day care and he cried—a lot. He hadn't been able to be soothed by feeding him, or cuddling him before she left, and eventually she had to leave him crying with the educators, who suggested that he would calm down after she was gone. She left in tears and cried all the way to work. Her son wasn't mobile yet, and she felt awful for leaving him, especially crying, when he was so little and so helpless. What if all the other kids just walked on him while he lay on the floor all day, she worried?

She called the day care when she got to work and they told her that her son had calmed down with a bottle soon after she had left, and was now on his educator's lap, playing with some blocks with another small baby. When she picked him up that afternoon, he was having some tummy time on the floor with another educator. Everything was fine.

Karen's son continued to cry when she left for a few weeks, and then after that it only happened sometimes. The educators assured her that he never cried for long. Overall, he seemed like the same happy, healthy baby he always was, and Karen started to get used to being back at work and her 'new normal'. The day-care educators started to feel familiar and a bit like an extended family to Karen and her son.

Her story: Maggie

Maggie always knew she wanted to stay home for at least a year after she had children. She was able to do so because her work offered extended maternity leave, on top of the government leave, and she was able to take her work leave at half-pay to double the amount of time off. Maggie loved spending her days with her daughter, but sometimes she struggled with the solitude during the day and felt lonely and disconnected from her friends and her world.

When her baby was younger, most of Maggie's friends worked or went to university and she didn't have family who lived nearby. Sometimes when her partner arrived home and told her about his day, she felt jealous that he had a 'whole life' outside of home, and she didn't feel like she did. She also felt jealous that when he got home, he had finished his job, while she was still going at hers, and would be all night—as she was the one who stayed home she took on all night wake-ups and feedings on her own.

Now that her baby is around eight months old and has started sleeping through the night and napping well, Maggie says she has found her flow and she has now gotten into a good routine with her days. She is really enjoying her time. She has started attending music lessons and swimming lessons with her baby, and has met some new friends that way, and is enjoying having some structure in her days. Maggie is still deciding whether she will go to work next year or continue to stay home, as she is enjoying it so much.

Her story: Fiona

Fiona is a new stay-at-home mum. She went back to work when her baby was six months old, but was struggling with her early morning starts, and not seeing her baby when she woke up. She left work when her baby was nine months old and has been home for three months now. She says that she sees many pros and many cons to the working mum versus the stay-at-home mum decision. She is enjoying the flexibility of her days with her daughter, and the fact that she can adjust her schedule as need be. She says she mostly enjoys the fact that many things can be done 'tomorrow' if she doesn't get to them today. However, she is missing being financially independent, and she says she feels guilty if she buys things for herself, such as a pair of new jeans, or even a cup of takeaway coffee. She also feels very lonely.

Although Fiona has a lot of mum friends, she feels isolated at home, and like 'mum is all I am these days'. She wonders if she would be friends with her mum friends if she wasn't a parent, or if that is all they have in common. Despite the cons she identifies, Fiona is happy with her decision. She says that she knows she will miss these days when they are gone, and that she will go back to work eventually—she thinks this will be when her daughter is in school—and she wants to 'soak all of it up' while she can. She says she feels extremely blessed that she has the option of staying home, and this is the first time she has discussed the cons because she knows a lot of people don't have the option of staying home, and she feels guilty for feeling this way.

Let's get practical

Whether you go back to work or not may be a choice you have to make, or it may be a given. If you do decide to go back to work, you will have some decisions to make, so here are some ideas that will hopefully help you with that.

Care options

If you work outside the home, you will need to decide what to do with your baby. What's that? Oh, you knew that already? Gosh, I thought I was being so helpful there. Yep, babies aren't great at staying home alone. These are some of your options:

- **Day-care centre:** These centres tend to be open long hours—ours is open from 6.15 a.m. to 6.15 p.m., for instance. If you work and commute within these hours, this can be a good option. In Australia there are standards that day-care centres need to meet, and they are assessed for these regularly. The ratio of child to educator is quite small, and it is all very safe and regulated. There are learning plans for each child, and parents are updated regularly on their child's learning and development. One of the biggest challenges of day-care centres is that, as we talked about, lots of kids can mean lots of germs and sicknesses.
- **Family day care:** These are run in someone's home. They are also regulated and standardised. They tend to be run by only one, sometimes two people, so the ratio of child

to educator is still small, but there are fewer kids overall, because there are fewer educators. (Good maths, hey!) It can be a very homey, cosy environment and some parents prefer this smaller, quieter environment for their child to a larger centre environment. Some kids may also do better in a quieter and less-stimulating environment, depending on their needs. There can also be less sickness in this type of arrangement, due to fewer kids, however, you may also need to find alternative care arrangements if your child's educator is sick, or on holidays.

- **In-home care:** Some parents opt for in-home care, such as nannies or au pairs. These carers may live with the family and provide childcare in return for accommodation, living costs and a small wage. Nannies may also live elsewhere and just come over during the day. Sometimes in-home carers may help with some housework as well. They can really become like a part of the family, and some parents love this option. It is usually more expensive than day care, though.

- **Family:** Some parents leave their babies with family members, often grandparents, while they go to work, or they may do this once a week or so and use other arrangements for the other days of the week. This is a fantastic option if it is available to your family, as grandparents are often thrilled to get some baby bonding time in.

- **Working in shifts:** If you have a partner, working shifts at separate times can eliminate (or reduce) the need for day care. This reduces costs and allows baby to stay with her parents all the time, but it also limits the amount of time that you see your partner, of course.

- **Work from home:** Some companies will allow this flexible work arrangement, as either part or all of your working week. However, many companies, even while allowing work-from-home scenarios, will stipulate that the parent must not have a child in their care during work hours, and in that case care arrangements will need to be made for the baby even if you are at home. If you can work from home while caring for your baby, this can be a wonderful, meaningful time. It has also been described as hectic, chaotic and 'like a zillion balls being juggled in the air at one time but no hands to catch even one of them' by one of the mums I spoke to. Working from home can seem like the ideal solution—no day-care fees, time with the baby, working in your jammies—but it is not an easy option in many ways!

Any of these options can be wonderful, and to work out which one is right for you, your baby and your family, I'd recommend having a chat with your partner if you have one and discussing any pros and cons that you can see.

Choosing day care

If you've decided to use a day-care centre or family day care, then you have even more decisions to make! Which one? Luckily, day-care providers are generally happy to show you around, bring baby in for a play, and answer any questions you may have. To choose, I would suggest:

- visiting lots of different places
- asking lots of questions
- investigating costs and what is included in these costs—meals, sunscreen, nappies, sheets, activities
- finding out what kinds of routine they follow, what kinds of activities they do
- finding out how they communicate with parents
- observing the interactions between the children and the carers
- paying attention to how you feel about the place: and listen to your mama instinct!

Ideas for working mums

Share the load—strategically

If you have a partner or someone at home to help you care for your baby, consider having a discussion around splitting up the tasks needed for the daily juggle that is a working-parent's life. Be strategic. For instance, if one partner doesn't mind cooking, have them take over that responsibility and do a weekly cook-up, where the other may not mind being the one to usually do the dishes, washing, or the day-care drop-off and pick-up. Another example is, one partner may take the lead with dressing, nappy changes, and soothing in the morning, and the other takes the lead at night. Consider your individual daily energy peaks and dips to divvy up the tasks. If you are usually rearing to go in the mornings, and your partner needs three cups of coffee to form a coherent sentence, you would probably be a good candidate for the morning, before work shift. If you are a night owl who finds it hard to wind down and relax after work, the afternoon shift may be for you.

Take a break

Take some time off. You now have two jobs. You have your paid job and your unpaid, at-home job. Though your at-home job is highly rewarding, and you probably wouldn't change it for anything, home is no longer a place to solely relax and unwind from work. It is the second shift. If it is at all possible, consider taking a morning or an afternoon a week off. If you are thinking this is highly unlikely, even impossible, I so get where you are coming from. It can feel impossible. In some situations, it is harder than others.

You may be a single mum or have a partner who is in the military, works long hours or works FIFO. If it isn't possible, it isn't possible. But if it is, if you have a partner or someone else you trust with your baby who is able and willing to relieve you, please consider taking some time for yourself regularly. It might only be a two-hour stretch, but if this is a regular occurrence, and something you can look forward to happening each week, I believe it will change your life.

If you are in a partnership, you may consider each choosing a time during the weekend where you get to do whatever you want, in the house or outside of the house. You might go for a swim, a nature walk, read, get a massage, or catch up with a friend. When it's your partner's turn, you might do something special to bond with your baby, like take them on a walk, or have a picnic in the backyard.

Planning and organisation

I was never a planning or organisation fan pre-kids. I'm still not really. I'd prefer to go with the flow, but I find some planning is so necessary, especially on work and day-care days. A cook-up on the weekend helps ensure day-care lunches and weeknight dinners are not too much of a stress during the week. Many mums told me that a cleaning schedule helps too, which I'm currently trying to implement. As an example, try doing a cook-up on Sunday, bathrooms on Saturday mornings, clean the fridge out and wash kitchen surfaces the night before whenever the bin goes out, floors on Friday night, and so on. (Party on, right!) This way, if you manage to keep on top of it all, you aren't stuck with a huge mountain of mess and cleaning to do. That can feel overwhelming, and make you want to throw things. (Well, this is what it does to me, anyway!) I'm so much more relaxed and ready to tackle the working week if my home is somewhat clean and organised. Don't get me wrong, my routine is not perfect, by any stretch of the imagination, but it helps.

Let go of guilt

Trust me, no one else is judging you as much as you are. Lots of people, bosses and day-care educators included, have been right where you are now. They understand the stresses of modern life, and they know that often you don't have much—read: any—control over either your work responsibilities or your parenting responsibilities. Most people get that you've got to do what you've got to do. Together with your employer and your child's carers, you will work it out, and this will be a much more pleasant experience for you if you can focus on the practical aspects of how to work it out and let go of the emotions and guilt surrounding something you absolutely cannot control.

Remember that regardless of whether you work outside of the home or not, you are still a full-time mum. You are still the one raising your child. Please know that your child recognises you as their mother, even if you are at work during the day, and to them, you are irreplaceable! I remember another mother asking me how I left my son at day care when he was five months old, stating that they could never let other people 'raise' their children. Day care is not raising your child, mama. That's all you.

Quality time

When time is limited, you start to value quality time over the quantity of your time. Though your time may be limited, you can connect with your baby in a meaningful way in a matter of minutes a day. Consider switching off technology, even just for fifteen minutes, and taking some time to just be with your baby—no agenda, no multitasking, just spending time together and reconnecting after a long day apart. If possible, you may do this in the morning as well. You can do what you must do in fifteen minutes time. For now, just be with each other.

Ideas for stay-at-home mums
Take a break

If one partner stays home, it is important that partners work together to give the stay-at-home parent a break from their full-time job. Though both partners are working all day, the stay-at-home parent has been working *in this job* all day. For their mental health, it is important that they can do something different, at least for a short while, each day. Partners need to work together to achieve this in the way that best suits their family. If there is no partner, consider talking to another family member or a friend about giving you a break.

Social connections

It is important for the stay-at-home mum to have a support network. Many mums spoke to me about feeling lonely, isolated or bored while at home. Those without strong support networks or friends at a similar stage of life were the most affected by this. You might want to join a playgroup or mothers' group, catch up with existing friends, or take part in a class, sport or hobby. Have someone take care of baby for a bit if there is no childcare available. Social connectivity is one of the strongest protective factors around postpartum mental health issues.

Value your identity

Remember, you are a whole, complete person outside of Mum. What are your goals, dreams and aspirations? Short-term, medium-term, long-term? Have a think about this. What would you like to achieve in the next month, the next year and the next five years? What could you be doing now to work towards those goals? You probably have some family goals, personal goals, relationship goals, spiritual goals, vocational goals or learning goals.

It is so important you remember these and take some time to focus on them regularly. Being a mum is important, fulfilling work. But it can be all-consuming. This can sometimes cause some resentment and a loss of personal identity. You became a mum, but you are still you, and you have the same needs as before. Don't forget you in the journey into motherhood!

A word on money

Many stay-at-home mums spoke to me about feeling they weren't contributing to the family because they weren't bringing in an income. Many felt guilty spending the smallest amount on themselves, even for practical things like new underwear. Firstly, you are contributing greatly. You are valued and worthy and you are doing a really tough job! It might be worth talking about this feeling with your partner if you have one. Most of the mums I have spoken with hadn't expressed to their partners that they felt this way about money, preferring to keep it to themselves. Consider having a frank discussion with your partner about both partners' roles and expectations around finances.

Reflection

- Do you think you would like to stay at home with your baby long-term, or are you planning on working outside the home? Are there any barriers to either of these options? Are they resolvable?
- How do you feel about the options you have?

- What is important to you in terms of care outside the home for your baby? I suggest writing these things down to discuss with potential care options.
- Are there barriers in the way of any of the practical tips we discussed for working mums or stay at home mums? How could you get around those barriers?

14

On Family Planning: When will we/will we have another?

As you get ready to blow out the candle on your baby's first cake, people inevitably start asking the question: 'Time for another?'

Many parents don't struggle with their family planning. They have a clear idea of how many kids they want, and that's what they try for. For a lot of other people, though, it's a struggle. Sometimes adding a subsequent child to your clan can be as big—or even bigger—a decision as having your first child! You are talking about changing the entire dynamic of a family, not just a couple. You must now factor in what's best for your child/children as well as for yourselves.

Lots of people get wrapped up and swept away in the excitement of pregnancy, birth and new babies. But having another baby is having another toddler, is having another school kid, is having another teenager, and another adult child. It's onesies and nappies, and it's also school fees and excursions and extra-curricular activities, and first cars and driving lessons, dating and weddings. I'm not saying that having more babies isn't the right decision for you—it may very well be that it is! I am saying it is important to consider whether you are deciding to do so *now* because you are ready to add another child to the family, not just another baby. Because as you now know, the baby stage flies by in a heartbeat!

As you settle into your new normal, the thought of adding another baby to the brood can be overwhelming. And thanks to those darn biological clocks, not making any decision can sometimes be a decision. For some people having more children is not an option for whatever reason. For others it is a struggle to decide whether to have another baby. As always, it's helpful to talk through the situations that can arise and affect these life-changing decisions in order to work out what's right for your family.

When partners don't agree

An additional challenge presents itself when partners disagree and have different ideas on what their ideal family looks like. This may have been discussed pre-relationship, but often hasn't. Or one—or both—partners may change their minds about how many children they would like, which we all have the right to do. It is an incredibly difficult, sensitive situation that might need some outside help to navigate.

It's not surprising that couples disagree on family size. Each person in a relationship is an individual. Couples don't meld into one person. They remain individuals with different wants, needs, temperaments, frustration tolerance, family backgrounds, personalities, preferences and opinions. This is okay and healthy.

Not only is it likely that you won't agree on everything, but this family planning business is extremely significant. It's going to affect your finances, lifestyles, energy levels and family composition. It's likely that whatever your stance, it's going to be a passionate and strong one, because the outcome will affect your whole life.

With most things, disagreements within a relationship are relatively easily to manage with good communication, creative problem-solving and compromise. But in this situation, there is no compromise. You can't half have another child, any more than you can have half another child. In this scenario, only one person is going to get their wish. It's important that couples seek to work through this issue together and remember that they are on the same team. They are not enemies and the ultimate goal for both is to have a happy, complete family.

Set aside an intentional time to discuss these issues. It's not a conversation to have over tacos in a busy restaurant or while driving with your baby crying in the backseat. Make time to listen with an open mind to each other's point of view. You probably both have reasons for wanting or not wanting to have another baby that the other person hasn't considered. Discussing the idea of another child also helps you both to process your own wants and needs.

After an intentional, honest, collaborative conversation, it may be that you still can't agree on the next steps in your family planning. This is okay. You are just being honest with each other. Leave the topic alone for a while and make a commitment to revisit the topic in another one, three or six months. Some couples unfortunately never agree on this decision. Sometimes partnerships do end over irreconcilable differences like this if one or both partners don't see a way past this issue, and they choose to pursue their family planning ideals outside of the current relationship. Most often, couples find a way through this challenge, though.

When there is no choice

Sometimes parents don't have the choice to have another child, perhaps due to relationship factors like divorce, or disagreement on family size. Secondary infertility can also be an issue. This is the inability to fall pregnant, or stay pregnant, after having previously given birth to a baby. This may happen for any number of reasons, but age, endometriosis, ovulation issues and impaired sperm production are thought to be common causes. Up to one in seven couples are found to struggle with secondary infertility and it's a type of grief that is frequently misunderstood by many people who haven't gone through it.

If you wish to have more children and for whatever reason this looks unlikely, it's an incredibly difficult process of grief and acceptance. It can also be quite a different experience to a couple struggling with primary infertility—as in, a couple with no children yet. There can be guilt about many things. For instance, parents can feel guilty that they are not providing their first child with a sibling, a playmate, or that if they eventually do they won't be close in age to their first. They may feel guilty because their partner is excited about the idea of a new baby. Parents can feel guilty for even feeling grief about secondary infertility, thinking they might be viewed as 'greedy' and 'ungrateful' because they have a child already and so many people don't.

Often other people can unknowingly contribute to this difficult experience. People, including strangers, feel more comfortable to comment on family size and planning with a couple who are already parents, and can minimise concerns with statements like, 'You know you can get pregnant' or, 'At least you have one already'. The couple struggling with secondary infertility can sometimes find it harder to gain support and understanding from their community. There can also be—probably unintentional—pressure from others. A couple of the women I spoke to who were struggling with secondary infertility said some of the most common things they were told by strangers upon hearing that they might not be having another child is, 'You wouldn't do that to your child, would you?' or, 'You'll change your mind, you'll see'. They confessed to me how incredibly difficult these types of statements are to hear.

Even though secondary infertility can be such a difficult and long process, ultimately the goal is to be able to accept and come to terms with the size of your family, and to actively choose to look for and enjoy the benefits that come with a family of your size, whatever it may be. The best gift that you can give to your child and to yourself is a content and happy life that focuses on what's good about where you are at and doesn't put conditions like 'when' or 'if only' on your happiness. Not that this is easy by any stretch of the imagination, but it's something to work towards, with outside help if you think that would be helpful.

In speaking to adolescents and adults who were only-children, lots of them loved their upbringing and only-child status. Unhappiness and dissatisfaction seems to arise when *parents* are not happy with having just one child, and they make this known to the child, usually subconsciously. I advise you to learn to accept your only-child status, if that's what ends up happening for you, regardless of whether this was by choice or not—I know, easier said than done when it is not a choice—and enjoy the many and varied benefits that come with the family of your size. Your child will most likely pick up on the attitude that his parents have towards his being the one child, so avoid making it a negative one. Of course, this advice stands however many children you end up having!

Her story: Julie

Julie and her husband had given a lot of thought to their family size before deciding to start trying for a baby, though they hadn't really discussed it before getting married. They discussed their career and personal goals, their temperaments—they are both introverted—their personalities, and their overall preferences, and realised that for both, one child was their dream. They were both passionate about their careers—John as a physiotherapist and Julie as a nurse—and both had goals of moving forward in those careers.

John and Julie also really wanted to travel and felt strongly that this needed to be a big part of their lives. As introverts, they knew that they functioned best when having frequent time alone and living in a peaceful and quiet environment—though that quiet part isn't working out too well now, as their bundle of joy is a rather wild, extroverted ten-year-old who loves having friends over all the time! For all these reasons and more besides, they decided a one-child family was best for them. They have remained certain in this decision and describe a content, happy and (usually) peaceful life with a well-adjusted, social and happy kid.

Their story: Fiona and Jodie

Fiona and Jodie were not sure how many children they wanted but agreed that they wanted a big family. Fiona remembers a fun, boisterous childhood with her four brothers and sisters. Jodie has only one sister, but always wanted more. Both have long harboured dreams of noisy Christmases, children playing together and a busy, active household. Before having kids, theirs was the house that friends would gather in, and they loved hospitality, socialising and having a house full of people. They were together for five years before they went down the IVF route and Fiona became pregnant with their first child. They knew they wanted another soon after and the next cycle of IVF produced twins! They were so happy with this, and they have certainly gotten their wish of a noisy and busy household. They aren't done though, planning on at least one more pregnancy.

Her story: Kathleen

Kathleen has a four-year-old daughter. She and her partner have been trying to conceive a second child for the past two-and-a-half years, as they were hoping to have two children close together in age. Kathleen has fallen pregnant once in that time but had an early miscarriage soon after first getting a positive pregnancy test—she estimates at around six weeks pregnant. She describes the sinking feeling in her tummy each month when her period comes. She talks about confusion, as she got pregnant easily with her daughter, who was a happy surprise not long after she and her partner started dating.

Kathleen says she now feels guilty, as she wanted her daughter to have a brother or sister to play with, and she fears that will never happen, or if it does, that they 'won't be friends' because they will have nothing in common being far apart in age. She is incredibly frustrated because her secondary infertility is unexplained, and so there is nothing that she, or anyone else including doctors, can do. She has considered the IVF route but at this stage it isn't affordable for their family. Kathleen and her partner are still trying to have another baby, but are considering whether they may stop trying, as they are unsure if they can live in this state of what Kathleen calls 'limbo'. She also feels it might be taking away from her relationship with her daughter.

Her story: Stacy

Stacy and her husband had not discussed the matter of children much before they got married quite young, at 24 and 25 years of age. They weren't sure whether they even wanted kids or not. As life went on, Stacy started to really want kids. She and her husband discussed it, and eventually decided to try to have a baby, which they did, around eighteen months later. He is now two years old. They are both very involved parents and love their son so much.

While Stacy feels she has more love to give to another child, and doesn't feel the family is yet complete, her husband doesn't think he has it in him to start again. He says he feels he has just enough energy, time and money now, and that having another might stretch him—and the family bank balance—to the point of not being able to provide the lifestyle he wants to for them. Stacy doesn't agree and is willing to make any number of sacrifices to make another child happen, such as foregoing holidays, moving to a cheaper house and budgeting strictly. Her partner feels that their family holidays and family house with the big backyard are things that will make their son's childhood happy and he doesn't want to make these sacrifices, plus he says there isn't any way to increase his energy levels or time and these are only likely to decrease with another child. They are at a stalemate but have been seeing a family counsellor to try to help them through this.

The counsellor has made the point that both have valid and thoughtfully considered points of view, that neither of them are acting out of selfishness, or fear or anxiety. They simply have different ideas around family planning. The counsellor said that they have a few choices: for one to accept the wishes of the other, and to become content with the idea of either having one child or two or more children and working together to make this scenario work for them, or to separate and pursue their family goals separately.

Hearing it this bluntly, both partners quickly realised that the last thing they wanted to do was separate, as they felt their marriage was the most important relationship in their life. They both decided that family size, though both had strong views on the matter, was not worth losing their relationship over. As it stands now, they have decided not to have another child for now, but to talk about it again in a year, when their son will be more independent and will be getting ready to go to kindergarten, to assess how they both feel at that stage.

Let's get practical

Think long-term

Often when we consider having a new baby, we consider just that: 'having a new baby'. We don't consider having a new toddler, school kid or teenager. An effective strategy is to look at the long-term, perhaps in five-year blocks of time. What do you hope for your family to look like in five years? Ten years? Fifteen years? Obvious as it sounds writing this, we can get swept up in the excitement of pregnancy and birth and forget that we are signing up for a new person, not just a new baby. We can tend to look at becoming pregnant and having a new baby as a goal, as something to be achieved, and if we are goal-oriented people, who always live for the next challenge, we can get so wrapped up in the next goal (pregnancy) that we forget to look beyond it. Conversely, we can let our fears around going through the 'newborn stage' again deter us from having another child, when that stage is, in the grand scheme of things, quite short.

Spend time in someone else's shoes

As a family, spend time with families of varying sizes. Spend time with other people's children. Offer to have a sleepover with your child's cousins or friends and see how it goes. Did you enjoy the noisier, busier, more unpredictable environment? How did you cope? How did your child cope? Could you see yourselves as a bigger family all the time? (Bonus for this strategy—you get to call on your family or friends to return the babysitting favour!)

Consider your finances

No one really likes to consider things like finances when it comes to their ideal family size; after all, a human life is price-less! Unfortunately, financial barriers to family size are a reality in our modern lives, and we do need to consider our finances in this decision. Obviously money is not everything and it doesn't buy happiness. (But it does buy stuff that makes you happy like chocolate and holidays, so that's the same thing isn't it?) It is an important thing to consider in family planning.

The cost of childcare and the cost of living in general places practical limits on what we can afford. Even if we can technically afford another child, we may not be able to afford it and still afford the things that are important to us. This might include private schooling, extra-curricular activities or frequent travel. We need to weigh up our options in this area. There isn't a right or wrong solution in this scenario, as people have different priorities, but these are things to consider.

Limit comparisons

Don't base your family planning on other people's families. When you begin hearing about friends and family having second (and third and fourth!) children, it can be easy to compare yourself, to become jealous or to become a bit confused or panicky. These are normal, but often fleeting feelings and it's important not to base important life decisions on what other people are doing. They are not you, and what's right for them may not be right for you.

Let go of the comparisons and the 'shoulds'. There is no formula for a happy family, or any perfect family size. There is only what is right for you. There might not even be one right choice for you—you could be completely happy as a family of two, three, or a family of ten! It's more about acceptance and what you make of what you have, rather than there being one answer for a happy family.

Ask questions—respectfully

Speak to and spend time with families of varying sizes. Speak to parents of only children, speak to adults who once were only children. Speak to adults who have siblings, and families who have multiple children. If you're all comfortable with it, voice your concerns, ask them what you want to know—make sure you ask them if they're okay to talk to you about this stuff first, and mention that you're just seeking information for your own planning purposes, and of course, ask your questions respectfully!

Reflection

- Have you given much thought to your ideal family size?
- If there is any disagreement between you and your partner regarding family size, have you set aside a time to intentionally discuss this? What would you like your partner to know about how you feel? What questions do you have for them? Consider taking these thoughts and questions with you when you discuss these issues, as it is easy to get flustered and forget them in the heat of the intense discussion.

The End

I want to sincerely thank you for sticking with me all the way through to the end of this book. I've absolutely loved the journey of connecting with mums from all around Australia and hearing their unique and touching stories.

Through the research I've done, and through talking to mums, I've identified common challenges women face when they first become parents. We are all unique though, and you might not have struggled in any of these areas! You might identify with all the challenges we've discussed, or some of them, or none of them. You might have struggled with an area that I haven't even touched on here.

Whatever your journey has been, I encourage you to talk to someone about it. You might choose to confide in a partner, or a friend, or a professional; depending on what suits you and your needs. As you work through the strategies and reflection questions in this book, if you feel that you have opened up a can of worms that you are having trouble closing on your own, the best gift you can give yourself and your baby is to find someone to help you reflect on this stuff and work through it. There is power and wisdom in recognising that we weren't meant to do some things alone.

The main message I wanted to convey throughout is grace. Well, grace and hope. I hope that the mums reading this will see that it is okay not to be okay. It's okay if the adjustment to motherhood is tough. New motherhood is an epic transition, an adjustment like no other. Yet, we sometimes forget that a mum is only newly born along with her first baby. Just as your baby wasn't a fully functional, independent human being straight out of the womb, neither are you expected to know everything, and immediately be able to cope with everything that motherhood entails. Becoming a mum is a gradual process. Give yourself some grace to learn and grow—take the pressure off. You do not have to be perfect at this—there is no such thing!

In the 'good old days', mothers had more of a village around them than we do now. Mothers were never supposed to learn all this stuff, and encounter all these challenges, alone. We still aren't, but modern society is set up in such a way that help is harder to access, and people are less likely to experience the village lifestyle than ever before. This leaves a lot on a new mum's shoulders. She often thinks she needs to provide everything a traditional village would by herself, or with a partner.

Additionally, there is a lot of pressure on modern-day mums. Social media allows us a front-row seat to the 'highlight reel' of other parents' lives. It also bombards us with—often conflicting—advice on things like feeding methods, sleeping practices, screen-time, parenting styles, disciplinary methods, and a million other things besides. We can be left feeling deflated, like nothing we are doing is 'enough' or 'right'; yet, we spend so much time and energy trying to get everything 'right' that we are increasingly distancing ourselves from the present moment with our children.

The secret is: there is no such thing as 'not enough' or 'right' if we love our children, we are safe, and we 'show up'—as in, respond to their needs in a gentle and positive manner. What this looks like may differ from person to person, depending on your temperament, personality type, support network, baby, and life-style, but you know yourself and your baby well enough to know what it looks like *for you and your baby*. Trust yourself. You've got this! Don't concern yourself with how others are doing it, or what other people think about your choices. If you are staying true to your values and your baby is loved and safe, all is well. We need to focus on raising our own families and disregard the many and varied opinions and experiences of those whose values may not align with ours, or to whom we might be comparing ourselves.

Babies are hard work. Very cute, but very hard work! It's astonishing that people so small can be that much work. When I had a new baby, I was always looking forward to the next stage. I thought life would be easier, and I would feel better once my son was sleeping better, once he was on solid food, once his reflux improved, once he could sit up, once he could crawl, once he could walk. (Seriously, I don't know what I was thinking with these last two—how did I think him being mobile would make life easier? I blame sleep deprivation!) I was placing conditions on my own happiness: *I will only be happy, and it will be much easier when and if . . . [insert next wish here].*

More seasoned mums would warn me about the 'terrible twos'. Later, the 'threenage years'. But wait, they would say, the threes are actually nothing compared to the 'fierce fours'! (Some people used a different 'F' word here!) Then the even-more seasoned mums would chuckle, 'Just *wait* until you hit the TEENAGE YEARS! Then you'll really know you're alive!' It seems that every age and stage has its challenges. But as my son nears four, I've yet to feel the way I did during the early postpartum period.

The postpartum period is unique. It's entering into a whole new role. It is going from 'me' to 'we', and you'll never be quite the same once you become Mum. Now that I'm past the adjustment stage, I adore being a mum, and it's really my favourite thing to do.

I am now passionate about helping new mums adjust to parenthood, because I struggled and now, as I connect with more and more mums, because I realise that *so many* mums struggle with it! It's a huge life change, and while some take to it like a duck to water, others need some time to just—you know, fully alter everything about their entire lives; for a while anyway. Rest assured, normality returns, albeit a 'new normal'. There is a light at the end of the tunnel!

For those of you who are trying to conceive, are pregnant, or are very new mums, I want to give you some hope. I know I have focused on the common challenges associated with the adjustment to motherhood. I did that because I've noticed that they don't get spoken about enough. Because research has consistently shown that realistic expectations are a positive and protective factor for a smoother transition through major life changes, I want you to be prepared for the common challenges that women face in the transition to motherhood.

What I haven't covered so much is the good stuff. I would do it all a million times over because, without the tough stuff, I wouldn't have gotten to do life with my absolute favourite person in the world: my son.

I know that as mums we sometimes feel like we are failures. We can feel as though the times we 'mess up' are going to screw our kids' lives up permanently. The good news is that kids are resilient. As long as we are there for them, we love them, and we keep trying, then getting up the next morning and trying again, they will be fine. More than fine—they will *thrive*.

A healthy and happy parent is a baby's most important asset. More than anything, they need us to love them. That's it. Sometimes to fully show love to our kids, we need to show ourselves a bit of self-care and love first. I truly hope everything I have spoken about has helped you to remember *you* in the journey to motherhood.

Perhaps you'd like to continue journaling your motherhood experience, now that you have gotten into the habit with your reflection questions. Writing can be incredibly cathartic, and something you can pass on if you want to. When my son was a baby, my mum gave me her diary from when I was a baby. This was such an incredible gift! I got to know my mum as a new mum, to learn about her struggles, her wins and, most importantly, how much she loved me.

Lastly, I just wanted to let you know that you're doing an amazing job. You are a caring and loving mum. You know how I know? Because you picked up this book. You care about your baby enough to actively prepare for parenting or maybe to work on any challenges you are facing now.

I wish you all the joy, happiness, love and full nights' sleeps (eventually) in the world.

Acknowledgements

I'd like to thank all of the amazing women I connected with while writing this book. Opening up about all of this required a beautiful vulnerability, and I have loved the experience of talking with you about your adjustment to parenthood. Thank you for being brave and allowing me to share your experiences in the hopes that they may help other women.

I would also love to thank my husband, Gavin. My writing this book sometimes required a lot of patience on your part, and I am truly so thankful for the way you supported me through this entire process. You helped me through any barriers in the way, including my own anxieties, and you made me a lot of cups of tea. Like, a lot.

My son, Eliah, thank you for just being you. You are a beautiful, gentle, funny, smart and cheeky boy, and I am so immensely grateful for you each and every day. I love you more than every colour in every rainbow.

Of course, this book would not exist if it wasn't for the incredible team at Allen & Unwin. Thank you to Claire Kingston, who saw some potential in this project and in me, and helped make a lifelong dream a reality; Kelly Fagan who held my hand through writing my first draft, making a scary undertaking feel a lot more manageable; and Samantha Kent, whose guidance, wisdom and support through the editing process were absolutely invaluable. I appreciate you all so much.

Notes

1. K. Lazurus & P.J. Rossouw, 'Mothers' Expectations of Parenthood: The impact of pre-natal expectations on self-esteem, depression, anxiety, and stress post-birth', *International Journal of Neuropsychotherapy*, 2015, vol. 3, no. 2, pp. 102–23.
2. R.J. Boorman, G.J. Devilly, J. Gamble, D.K. Creedy & J. Fenwick, 'Childbirth and the Criteria for Traumatic Events', *Midwifery*, 2014, vol. 30, no. 2, pp. 255–61. <https://doi.org/10.1016/j.midw.2013.03.001>
3. I.S. Polachek, L.H. Harari, M. Baum & R.D. Strous, 'Postpartum Post-traumatic Stress Disorder Symptoms: The uninvited birth companion', *Israeli Medical Association*, 2012, vol. 14, no. 6, pp. 347–53.
4. E. Abraham, T. Hendler, I. Shapira-Lichter, Y. Kanat-Maymon, O. Zagoory-Sharon & R. Feldman, 'Father's Brain is Sensitive to Childcare Experiences', *Proceedings of the National Academy of Sciences in the United States of America*, 2014, vol. 111, no. 27, pp. 9792–7. <https://doi.org/10.1073/pnas.1402569111>
5. J.P. Sacher, V. Rekkas, A.A. Wilson, S. Houle, L. Romano, J. Hamidi, I.E. Rusjan, D.E. Stewart & J.H. Meyer, 'Relationship

of Monoamine Oxidase: A distribution volume to postpartum depression and postpartum crying', *Neuropsychopharmacology*, 2015, vol. 40, no. 2, pp. 429–35. <https://doi.org/10.1038/npp.2014.190>

6. S. Shepherd, 'How to Cope with Postpartum "Baby Blues"—From a Clinical Psychologist', <www.mother.ly/life/how-to-cope-with-postpartum-baby-blues-from-a-clinical-psychologist>

7. V. Fallon, S. Komnimou, K.M. Bennett, J.C.G. Halford & J.A. Harrold, 'The Emotional and Practical Experiences of Formula-feeding Mothers', *Maternal & Child Nutrition*, 2016, vol. 13, no. 3. <https://doi.org/10.1111/mcn.12392>

8. C.G. Colen & D.M. Ramey, 'Is Breast Truly Best? Estimating the effects of breastfeeding on long-term child health and wellbeing in the United States using sibling comparisons', *Social Science and Medicine*, 2014, vol. 109, pp. 55–65. <https://doi.org/10.1016/j.socscimed.2014.01.027>

9. Colen & Ramey, 'Is Breast Truly best?'

10. R. Patel, E. Oken, N. Bogdanovich, L. Matush, Z. Sevkovskaya, B. Chalmers, E.D. Hodnett, K. Vilchuck, M.S. Kramer & R.M. Martin, 'Cohort Profile: The promotion of breastfeeding intervention trial (PROBIT)', *International Journal of Epidemiology*, 2013, vol. 43, no. 3, pp. 679–90. <https://doi.org/10.1093/ije/dyt003>

11. K.L. Armstrong, R.A. Quinn & M.R. Dadds, 'The Sleep Patterns of Normal Children', *The Medical Journal of Australia*, 1994, vol. 161, pp. 202–6.

12. V.S. Gelman, M.K. Jory & P.G. Macris, 'Personality Factors in Mothers of Children Who Wake at Night', *Australian Journal of Psychology*, 2011, vol. 50, no. 1, pp. 25–8. <https://doi.org/10.1080/00049539808257527>

13. E.S. Grossman & T. Rosenbloom, 'Perceived Level of Performance Impairment Caused by Alcohol and Restricted Sleep', *Traffic Psychology and Behaviour*, 2016, vol. 41, pp. 113–23. <https://doi.org/10.1016/j.trf.2016.06.002>

14. S. Nowakowski, J. Meers & E. Heimback, 'Sleep and Women's Health', *Sleep Medicine Research*, 2013, vol. 4, no. 1, pp. 1–22.

15. I originally wrote about emotional eating in the newborn stage for an online parenting magazine called www.parent.co: S. Shepherd, 'The Link Between Emotional Eating and Parenthood', www.mother.ly, 2017. <www.mother.ly/parenting/link-emotional-eating-parenthood>

16. G.S. Bruin, *The Language of Recovery: Understanding and treating addiction*, CreateSpace Independent Publishing Platform: Amazon, 2010, Chapter 1.

17. Australian Bureau of Statistics, *National Survey of Mental Health and Wellbeing: Summary of results, 2007*, Cat. No. (4326.0), Canberra: ABS, 2008.

18. N. Highet, *Communication Around Perinatal Emotional and Mental Health: The rationale for a new approach to positioning information outside of a mental health context*, <https://cope.org.au/wp-content/uploads/2016/02/COPE-Community-awareness-Research-Summary.pdf>, 2015.

19. ABS, *National Survey of Mental Health and Wellbeing*.

20. Highet, *Communication Around Perinatal Emotional and Mental Health*.

21. B. Laditan, 'How to be a mum in 2017', <www.thehonesttoddler.com>, retrieved 2019.

22. J. Horan-Smith & E. Gullone, 'Screening an Australian Community Sample for Risk of Postnatal Depression, *Australian Psychologist*, 2018, vol. 33, no. 2, pp. 138–42. <https://doi.org/10.1080/00050069808257395>

23. American Psychiatric Association, *Diagnostic and Statistical Manual of Mental Disorders* (5th edition), Arlington, VA: American Psychiatric Publishing, 2013, pp. 160–86.

24. T.W. Kjaer, C. Bertelsen, P. Piccini, D. Brooks, J. Alving & H.C. Lou, 'Increased Dopamine Tone During Meditation-induced Change of Consciousness', *Cognitive Brain Research*, 2002, vol. 13, no. 2, pp. 255–9. <https://doi.org/10.1016/S0926-6410(01)00106-9>

25. A.T. Beck, *Cognitive Therapy and the Emotional Disorders*, Oxford, England: International Universities Press, 1976.

26. D.D. Burns, *Feeling Good: The new mood therapy*, New York, NY: Penguin Books, 1981.

27. Perinatal Anxiety and Depression Australia, <www.panda.org.au>.

28. L.S. Leach, C. Poyser & K. Fairweather-Schmidt, 'Maternal Perinatal Anxiety: A review of prevalence and correlates', *Clinical Psychologist*, 2017, vol. 21, pp. 4–19. <https://doi.org/10.1111/cp.12058>

29. B. Figueiredo & A. Conde, 'Anxiety and Depression in Women and Men from Early Pregnancy to 3 Months Postpartum', *Archives of Womens' Mental Health*, 2011, vol. 14, no. 3, pp. 247–55. <https://doi.org/10.1007/S00737-011-0217-3>

30. American Psychiatric Association, *Diagnostic and Statistical Manual of Mental Disorders*, pp. 189–242.

31. I.M. Paul, D.S. Downs, E.W. Schaefer, J.S. Beiler & C.S. Weisman, 'Postpartum Anxiety and Maternal–Infant Health Outcomes,' *Pediatrics*, 2013, vol. 131, no. 4, pp. 1218–24. <https://doi.org/10.1542/peds.2012-2147>

32. C.F. Zambaldi, A. Cantilino, A.C. Montenegro, J.A. Paes, T.L. de Albuquerque & E.B. Sougey, 'Post-partum Obsessive-Compulsive Disorder: Prevalence and clinical characteristics', *Comprehensive*

Psychiatry, 2009, vol. 50, no. 6, pp. 503–9. <https://doi.org/10.1016/j.comppsych.2008.11.014>

33. J.R. Britton, 'Infant Temperament and Maternal Anxiety and Depressed Mood in the Early Postpartum Period', *Women and Health*, 2011, vol. 51, no. 1, pp. 55–71. <https://doi.org/10.1080/03630242.2011.540741>

34. P.D. Pilkington, T.A. Whelan & L.C. Milne, 'A Review of Partner-inclusive Interventions for Preventing Postnatal Depression and Anxiety', *Clinical Psychologist*, 2015, vol. 19, no. 2, pp. 63–75. <https://doi.org/10.1111/cp.12054>

35. S. Shapiro, J. Gottman & S. Carrere, 'The Baby and The Marriage: Identifying factors that buffer against decline in marital satisfaction after the first baby arrives', *Journal of Family Psychology*, 2000, vol. 14, no. 1, pp. 59–70. <https://doi.org/10.1037//0893-3200.14.1.59>

36. J.M. Gottman & N. Silver, *The Seven Principles for Making Marriage Work*, New York: Three Rivers Press, 1999.

37. P. Fomby & A.J. Cherlin, 'Family Instability and Child Wellbeing', *American Sociological Review*, 2007, vol. 72, pp. 181–204. <https://doi.org/10.1177/000312240707200203>.

38. G.C. Rubin, *The Happiness Project: Or why I spent a year trying to sing in the morning, clean my closets, fight right, read Aristotle, and generally have more fun*, Toronto: HarperCollins, 2011.

39. C. Sok, J.N. Sanders, H.M. Saltzman & D.K. Turok, 'Sexual Behaviour, Satisfaction, and Contraceptive Use Among Post-partum Women', *Journal of Midwifery & Women's Health*, 2016, vol. 61, no. 2, pp. 158–65. <https://doi.org/10.1111/jmwh.12409>

40. J.E. Fehniger, J.S. Brown, J.M. Creasman, S.K. Van Dan Eeden, D.H. Thorn, L.L. Subak & A.J. Huang, 'Childbirth and Female

Sexual Function Later in Life', *Obstetrics and Gynecology*, 2013, vol. 122, no. 5, pp. 988–97. <https://doi.org/10.1097/AOG.0b013e3182a7f3fc>

41. S. Pertot, 'Postpartum Loss of Sexual Desire and Enjoyment', *Australian Journal of Psychology*, 1981, vol. 33, no. 1, pp. 11–18.

42. G.D. Chapman, *The 5 Love Languages: The secret to love that lasts*, Chicago: Northfield Pub, 2010, pp. 37–120.

43. C.H. Ou & W. Hall, 'Anger in the Context of Postnatal Depression: An integrative review', *Birth*, 2018, pp. 1–11. <https://doi.org/10.1111/birt.12356>

44. University of British Columbia, 'Anger Overlooked as a Feature of Postnatal Mood Disorders', *Science Daily*, 26 June 2018, <www.sciencedaily.com/releases/2018/06/180626113415.htm>, retrieved 16 August 2018.

45. C.T. Beck, 'Postpartum Depressed Mothers' Experiences Interacting with their Children, *Nurse Research*, 1996, vol. 45, pp. 98–104 (cited in Ou & Hall, 'Anger in the Context of Postnatal Depression').

46. B.J. Bushman, 'Does Venting Anger Feed or Extinguish the Flame? Catharsis, rumination, distraction, anger, and aggressive responding', *Personality and Social Psychology Bulletin*, 2002, vol. 28, no. 6, pp. 724–31.

47. L. Festinger, *A Theory of Cognitive Dissonance*, California, USA: Stanford University Press, 1957.

48. Australian Bureau of Statistics, *Labour Force Australia: Labour force status and other characteristics of families,* ABS, Cat. No. 6224.0, 2017, <www.abs.gov.au/AUSSTATS/abs@.nsf/mf/6224.0.55.001>, retrieved 20 December 2018.

49. Australian Bureau of Statistics, *Labour Force Australia.*

50. J. Rose, 'Never Enough Hours in the day: Employed mothers' perceptions of time pressure', *Australian Journal of Social Issues*, 2017, vol. 52, no. 2, pp. 116–30. <https://doi.org/10.1002/ajs4.2>

Index